Salad Recipe Cookbook, Plant Based Diet Cookbook, Binge Eating Overcome Overeating, Fitness Nutrition & Bodyweight Training

© Copyright 2018 by Charlie Mason - All rights reserved.

The follow Book is reproduced below with the goal of providing information that is as accurate and reliable as possible. Regardless, purchasing this Book can be seen as consent to the fact that both the publisher and the author of this book are in no way experts on the topics discussed within and that any recommendations or suggestions that are made herein are for entertainment purposes only. Professionals should be consulted as needed prior to undertaking any of the action endorsed herein.

This declaration is deemed fair and valid by both the American Bar Association and the Committee of Publishers Association and is legally binding throughout the United States.

Furthermore, the transmission, duplication or reproduction of any of the following work including specific information will be considered an illegal act irrespective of if it is done electronically or in print. This extends to creating a secondary or tertiary copy of the work or a recorded copy and is only allowed with express written consent from the Publisher. All additional right reserved.

The information in the following pages is broadly considered to be a truthful and accurate account of facts and as such any inattention, use or misuse of the information in question by the reader will render any resulting actions solely under their purview. There are no scenarios in which the publisher or the original author of this work can be in any fashion deemed liable for any hardship or damages that may befall them after undertaking information described herein.

Additionally, the information in the following pages is intended only for informational purposes and should thus be thought of as universal. As befitting its nature, it is presented without assurance regarding its prolonged validity or interim quality. Trademarks that are mentioned are done without written consent and can in no way be considered an endorsement from the trademark holder.

BONUS:

As a way of saying thank you, I have laid out 3 FREE Easy Cookbooks to get yourself onto the path that leads to the fitter, healthier you!

[Click here to Get 3 FREE Cookbooks on Health, Fitness & Dieting Instantly!](#)

Table of Contents

The Complete Salad Recipe Cookbook 8
    Chapter 1: Traditional Salad Recipes 9
    Chapter 2: Quick and Easy Salad Recipes 16
    Chapter 3: Group Salad Recipes 23
    Chapter 4: Salads for the Entire Family 31
    Chapter 5: Lunch Salads 40
    Conclusion 47

THE COMPLETE PLANT-BASED COOKBOOK 48
    Portobello Bruschetta 50
    Baked Vegetable Foil Packs 1
    Sweet Potato and Black Bean Tacos 2
    Avocado and White Bean Sandwich 3
    Veggie-Loaded Rice Bowls 4
    Hummus Vegetable Wrap 5
    Zucchini Noodle Pasta with Avocado Pesto 6
    Turmeric Roasted Potatoes and Asparagus 7
    Vegan Zucchini Boats 8
    Tomato Basil Soup 10
    Thai Peanut Tofu with Sautéed Vegetables 11
    Dark Chocolate Covered Bananas 13
    No-Bake Peanut Butter Cookies Drizzled with Dark Chocolate .. 14
    Vegan Pineapple Ice Cream 15
    Matcha & Coconut Power Bars 16
    Cashew Whipped Cream with Berries 17
    Vegan Dark Chocolate Mint Mousse 18
    Raw Chocolate Brownies 19

Banana Almond Chia Pudding 20
Chocolate Chip Energy Bits 21
Almond Butter Apple Slices 22
No-Bake Chocolate Cookie Dough Bars 23
Triple Berry Ice Cream 24
Ginger Cookies with Cashew Vanilla Icing 25
Blueberry Almond Smoothie 26
Green Mango Protein Smoothie 27
Strawberry Banana Smoothie 28
Hemp Oatmeal Chocolate Smoothie 29
Vanilla Cashew Smoothie 30
Lavender Blueberry Smoothie 31
Avocado Kale & Raspberry Smoothie 32
Tropical Acai Smoothie 33
Green Avocado Smoothie 34
Superfood Smoothie 35
Energizing Kale Smoothie 36
Refreshing Pineapple Protein Smoothie 37
Purple Antioxidant Smoothie 38
Mandarin Kale Salad with Sweet Tahini Dressing 40
Thai Zucchini Noodle Salad 41
Tomato Avocado Onion Salad 42
Watermelon & Jasmine Rice Salad 43
Mango Black Bean Salad 44
Red Apple & Kale Salad 45
Cauliflower & Chickpea Salad 46
Strawberry Mango and Pineapple Tacos 47
Rainbow Beet Salad 48

Walnut & Pear Salad with Lemon Poppy Seed Dressing 49
White Bean & Asparagus Salad 50
3 Bean Salad with Roasted Sweet Potatoes 51

Binge Eating 54

Introduction 55
Chapter 1: Identifying and Overcoming Causes of Bingeing 56
Chapter 2: Manage your food 60
Chapter 4: Create Sustainable Eating and Living Habits 68
Chapter 5: Self-Acceptance and Avoiding Relapse 72
Conclusion 76

Fitness Nutrition: 78

Introduction 79
Chapter 1: 81
Chapter 2: Abs, Back, and Biceps 84
Chapter 3: Hamstrings, Quads, and Calves 88
Chapter 4: Cardio HIIT 91
Chapter 5: Abs 95
Chapter 6: Obliques 98
Chapter 7: Outer and Inner Thighs 100
Chapter 8: Butt 102
Chapter 9: Back 103
Chapter 10: Nutrition and Fitness go Hand in Hand 105
Chapter 11: Top SEVEN Delicious Plant-based Recipes 107
Conclusion 113

The Complete Bodyweight Training: 114

Introduction 115
Chapter 1: Why Bodyweight Training Kicks Butt 117
Chapter 2: Upper Body Workouts 120

Chapter 3: Lower Body Workouts 129
Chapter 4: Core Training.. 137
Conclusion 144

The Complete Salad Recipe Cookbook

Chapter 1: Traditional Salad Recipes

Classic three bean salad

Total Prep & Cooking Time: 9 hours
Yields: 6 Servings

What to Use

- Pepper (as desired)
- Salt (as desired)
- Green beans (16 oz. drained)
- White sugar (.25 c)
- Vegetable oil (.5 c)
- Vinegar (.5 c)
- Pimento peppers (4 oz. drained, chopped)
- Green bell pepper (1 c chopped)
- Celery (1 c chopped)
- Onion (1 c chopped)
- Red kidney beans (16 oz. drained)
- Yellow wax beans (16 oz. drained)
- Green beans (16 oz. drained)

What to Do

- In a serving bowl, combine the green bell pepper, celery, onion, kidney beans, yellow wax beans, pimento peppers and green beans and mix well to combine thoroughly.
- In a saucepan, combine the pepper, salt, sugar oil and vinegar and mix well before placing the saucepan on the stove over a burner turned to a high heat and allow it boil, stirring throughout so the sugar dissolves.

- Toss salad with dressing to coat before placing the serving dish in the refrigerator for at least 8 hours to allow flavors to properly mix.

Classic Israeli cucumber and tomato salad

Total Prep & Cooking Time: 20 minutes
Yields: 6 Servings

What to Use

- Pepper (as desired)
- Salt (as desired)
- Lemon juice (2 T)
- Olive oil (.5 c)
- Garlic (2 T chopped)
- Red bell pepper (1 diced, seeded)
- Purple onion (.5 diced)
- Roma tomatoes (4 diced, seeded)
- English cucumbers (4 diced)

What to Do

- Combine the pepper, salt, lemon juice and olive oil together in a small bowl and mix well to combine thoroughly.
- Add the English cucumbers, Roma tomatoes, purple onion, red bell pepper and chopped garlic to a serving bowl and mix well.
- Toss with dressing to ensure it is fully coated.

Classic seven-layer salad

Total Prep & Cooking Time: 50 minutes
Yields: 8 Servings

What to Use

- Pepper (as desired)
- Salt (as desired)
- Bacon (.5 c cooked, crumbled)
- Water chestnuts (4 oz. drained, sliced)
- Peas (10 oz. frozen, thawed)
- Black olives (6 oz. drained, sliced)
- Roma tomatoes (to taste, chopped)
- Iceberg lettuce (4 c torn)
- Mayonnaise (1.25 c)
- Cheddar cheese (2 c shredded)

What to Do

- In a small bowl, combine the mayonnaise and cheddar cheese and combine thoroughly.
- In a glass serving bowl, form the lettuce into a firm layer on the bottom of the bowl. Top that layer with a layer of tomatoes, followed by a layer of black olive, then a layer of peas and then finally a layer of water chestnuts. Top with a layer of cheddar cheese and then finish it off with a layer of bacon.
- Top the bacon layer with a firm layer of plastic wrap and then place the salad in the refrigerator for at least 30 minutes.
- Serve chilled.

Classic cucumber salad

Total Prep & Cooking Time: 135 minutes
Yields: 6 Servings

What to Use

- Pepper (as desired)
- Salt (as desired)
- White onion (1 sliced into rings)
- Tomatoes (3 wedged)
- Cucumbers (3 sliced, peeled)
- Sugar (.25 c)
- Vegetable oil (.25 c)
- White vinegar (.5 c distilled)
- Water (1 c)

What to Do

- In a large serving bowl, whisk together the pepper, salt, sugar, oil, vinegar and water before adding in the onion, tomatoes and cucumber and tossing to coat.
- Cover the serving bowl with plastic wrap and let it chill in the refrigerator for at least two hours prior to serving.

Classic German potato salad

Total Prep & Cooking Time: 4 hours
Yields: 10 Servings

What to Use

- Pepper (as desired)
- Salt (as desired)
- Sugar (2 T)

- Water (.5 c)
- White vinegar (1 c)
- Garlic (4 cloves minced)
- Sweet onions (2 diced)
- Bacon (1 lb.)
- Red potatoes (5 lbs. diced)

What to Do

- Add the potatoes to a pot before filling the pot with water so the potatoes are completely covered. Season as desired before placing the pot on the stove over a burner turned to a high heat. Allow the water to boil before reducing the heat to low/medium and letting the potatoes simmer for about 20 minutes or until they are nice and tender. Drain the potatoes before adding them to a slow cooker.
- Add the bacon to a skillet before placing the skillet on the stove over a burner turned to a high/medium heat and letting it cook about 10 minutes. Crumble the bacon and add it to the potatoes.
- Reheat the skillet to a medium heat, while retaining the bacon grease. Add in the onions and let them cook 5 minutes before adding in the garlic and cooking 2 more minutes. Add the results to the slow cooker.
- In a small bowl, mix together the salt, sugar, water and vinegar and combine thoroughly before adding it to the top of the slow cooker and mixing well.
- Allow the slow cooker to cook, covered, for 4 hours on a low heat.

Classic Greek salad

Total Prep & Cooking Time: 10 minutes
Yields: 8 Servings

What to Use

- Pepper (as desired)
- Salt (as desired)
- Red onion (.5 sliced)
- Sun-dried tomatoes (.3 c drained, oil reserved)
- Roma tomatoes (3 c diced)
- Black olives (1 c pitted, sliced)
- Feta cheese (1.5 c crumbled)
- Cucumbers (3 sliced, seeded)

What to Do

- Combine all of the ingredients in a serving bowl and mix well.
- Toss with dressing as desired.
- Cover the serving bowl with plastic wrap and chill prior to serving.

Classic Mediterranean salad

Total Prep & Cooking Time: 50 minutes
Yields: 4 Servings

What to Use

- Pepper (as desired)
- Salt (as desired)
- Lemon (1 zested)
- Oregano (2 tsp. dried)

- Garlic (2 cloves minced)
- White vinegar (1 T)
- Parsley (2 T)
- Extra-virgin olive oil (.25 c)
- Lemons (2 juiced)
- Zucchini (3 spiralized)
- Kalamata olive (.5 c pitted, halved)
- Cherry tomatoes (1 c halved)
- Artichoke hearts (10 oz. chopped, drained)

What to Do

- Combine the zucchini, olives, tomatoes and artichoke hearts in a serving bowl and mix well.
- In a separate bowl, combine the pepper, salt, lemon zest, oregano, garlic, vinegar, parsley, olive oil and lemon juice and mix well to combine thoroughly.
- Add the dressing to the salad and toss to coat.
- Top the zucchini with feta cheese prior to serving.

Chapter 2: Quick and Easy Salad Recipes

Chef Salad

Total Prep & Cooking Time: 15 minutes
Yields: 4 Servings

What to Use

- Pepper (as desired)
- Salt (as desired)
- Monterey Jack cheese (4 oz. shredded)
- Radishes (6 sliced thin)
- Avocado (1 pitted, sliced)
- Boston lettuce (1 head large)
- Honey (1 T)
- Sour cream (.3 c)
- Carrots (4 sliced)
- Alfalfa sprouts (1 c)
- Roasted turkey (1 lb. sliced, torn)
- Apple cider vinegar (2 T)
- Buttermilk (.3 c low-fat)

What to Do

- Combine the cheese, carrots, radishes, sprouts, avocado, turkey and lettuce in a serving bowl and mix well.
- In a small separate bowl combine the pepper, salt, honey, vinegar, sour cream and buttermilk and whisk well.
- Toss with dressing as desired prior to serving.

Thai Salad

Total Prep & Cooking Time: 20 minutes
Yields: 4 Servings

What to Use

- Pepper (as desired)
- Salt (as desired)
- English cucumber (1 halved, peeled, chopped)
- Serrano chili (chopped)
- Lime juice (.25 c)
- Safflower oil (2 T)
- Mint leaves (1 handful chopped)
- Brown sugar (2 tsp.)
- Fish sauce (2 T)
- Red onion (.5 sliced thin)
- Napa cabbage (1 head)
- Pork chops (4)

What to Do

- Place a skillet over a burner turned to a high heat and let it heat up for 5 minutes before adding half of the cabbage and letting it cook about 3 minutes, flipping in the middle.
- Remove the cabbage from the skillet, add 1 T oil and then add in the pork and cook each side about 2 minutes until its internal temperature is at least 140 degrees F.
- Remove the pork from the skillet and slice it once it has cooled slightly and combine all of the ingredients in a serving dish and toss to combine before dividing evenly among the plates with the cabbage on the bottom.

Chicken salad with green beans and cherries

Total Prep & Cooking Time: 15 minutes
Yields: 4 Servings

What to Use

- Pepper (as desired)
- Salt (as desired)
- Cherries (.3 c dried)
- Arugula (5 oz.)
- Apricot jam (1 T)
- Green beans (.5 lb. trimmed)
- Chicken breast cutlets (1 lb.)
- Almonds (.25 c sliced)
- Radicchio (1 head, shredded, cored)
- Dijon mustard (1 T)
- Red wine vinegar (3 T)
- Olive oil (3T)

What to Do

- Add 1 T oil to a skillet before placing it on a burner turned to a high heat before adding in the seasoned chicken and cooking it about 1.5 minutes per side until it reaches an internal temperature of 165 degrees F. Remove the chicken from the skillet and slice it when cool.
- Add 2 inches slated water to a saucepan and place it on a burner turned to a high heat and allow it to boil before adding in the green beans and letting them cook about 4 minutes. Rinse under cold water and drain.
- In a small bowl, combine 2 T oil, mustard, jam and vinegar and whisk well before seasoning as desired
- Add the remaining ingredients to a serving bowl and toss well.

- Plate the salad, top with the chicken and then the dressing prior to serving.

Steak salad

Total Prep & Cooking Time: 20 minutes
Yields: 4 Servings

What to Use

- Pepper (as desired)
- Salt (as desired)
- Carrots (3 sliced)
- Red leaf lettuce (1 head torn)
- Dijon mustard (1 T)
- Olive oil (2 T)
- Radishes (8 quartered)
- Garlic (1 clove minced)
- White wine vinegar (2 T)
- Snap peas (8 oz. halved, steamed)
- Skirt steak (1 lb. halved)

What to Do

- Heat your broiler before placing the steak on top of a baking sheet lined with tinfoil (seasoned as desired) and broiling the steak for 4 minutes. Remove the steak from the broil and tent it in the tinfoil to keep it warm.
- Combine the garlic, mustard, vinegar and oil and whisk well to combine thoroughly. Toss the lettuce using half the dressing.
- Slice the steak and place it and the remaining ingredients on top of the tossed salad. Top with dressing prior to serving.

Chicken salad with pistachios and feta

Total Prep & Cooking Time: 20 minutes
Yields: 4 Servings

What to Use

- Pepper (as desired)
- Salt (as desired)
- Feta (4 oz. crumbled)
- Parsley (.5 c)
- Coriander (1 tsp.)
- Olive oil (.25 c + 1 T)
- Navel oranges (2 halved, sliced thin)
- Scallions (1 bunch sliced thin)
- Romaine lettuce (1 head chopped)
- Chicken cutlets (1 lb.)
- White wine vinegar (.25 c)
- Pistachios (.5 c)

What to Do

- Add the pistachios to a skillet before placing the skillet on a burner turned to a medium heat. All them to cook for 7 minutes, regularly stirring.
- Once they have cooled place them in a bowl and whisk in vinegar, .25 c oil, salt and pepper and mix well.
- Add the rest of the of the oil to the skillet before seasoning the chicken and cooking it about 2 minutes per side or until its internal temperature reaches 165 degrees F. Slice the chicken once it has cooled.
- Combine the scallions, parsley, lettuce and pistachios with the dressing and toss well. Plate the salad before topping with oranges, feta and chicken.

Spinach salad with salmon

Total Prep & Cooking Time: 15 minutes
Yields: 4 Servings

What to Use

- Pepper (as desired)
- Salt (as desired)
- Pecans (.25 c)
- Grape tomatoes (1 pint halved)
- Balsamic vinaigrette (.25 c)
- Goat cheese (.75 c crumbled)
- Baby spinach (10 oz.)
- Salmon fillet (4 skin removed)

What to Do

- Place the salmon on a lined baking sheet and season as desired before broiling the fish about 7 minutes. Flake the fish once it has cooled.
- Combine the remaining ingredients together and plate before topping with the fish, pecans and goat cheese. Drizzle with vinaigrette prior to serving.

Zucchini salad with chicken

Total Prep & Cooking Time: 30 minutes
Yields: 4 Servings

What to Use

- Pepper (as desired)
- Salt (as desired)
- Mint (.25 c chopped)
- Pecans (.75 c chopped)
- Spinach (8 oz. chopped)
- Zucchini (1.25 lbs. sliced thin)
- Lemon juice (.25 c)
- Parmesan cheese (.25 c grated)
- Red onion (.5 sliced thin)
- Chicken breast (1 lb.)
- Olive oil (.25 c + 1 T)

What to Do

- Combine the lemon juice and .25 c oil in a serving bowl and mix well before adding in the zucchini and tossing to coat. Allow it to remain in the mixture while the chicken cooks.
- Add the rest of the oil to a skillet before placing the skillet on a burner set to a medium heat. Season the chicken as desired before adding it to the skillet and letting it cook until it reaches an internal temperature of 165 degrees.
- Add all of the ingredients to the serving bowl and toss well prior to serving.

Chapter 3: Group Salad Recipes

Zucchini salad with Arugula

Total Prep & Cooking Time: 20 minutes
Yields: 10 Servings

What to Use

- Pepper (as desired)
- Salt (as desired)
- Basil leaves (25)
- Arugula (5 oz.)
- Balsamic vinaigrette (.25 c + 1 T)
- Grape tomatoes (10 oz.)
- Mozzarella cheese (2.5 lbs. cubed)
- Zucchini (5 spiralized)

What to Do

- Add the vinaigrette, tomatoes, mozzarella and zucchini in a serving bowl and mix well. Place in the refrigerator until you are ready to serve.
- Prior to serving mix in the basil and arugula.

Caesar salad sandwich

Total Prep & Cooking Time: 25 minutes
Yields: 10 Servings

What to Use

- Pepper (as desired)
- Salt (as desired)
- Parmesan cheese (1.25 c shredded)
- Caesar salad dressing (2.5 c)
- Romaine lettuce (2.5 heads quartered)
- Tomatoes (2.5 halved)
- Garlic (5 cloves halved)
- Olive oil (.5 c + 2 T)
- Baguettes (2.5)

What to Do

- Prepare your grill to a low temperature and ensure the grate is oiled.
- Slice baguettes in quarters and brush using olive oil.
- Grill the baguette pieces for about 2 minutes per side. Rub the bread with tomatoes and garlic and set it aside.
- Use the rest of the olive oil to brush the romaine lettuce and then grill it for about 2 minutes per side. Season with salt and set it aside.
- Place the lettuce on top of the baguette and top with Caesar dressing and Parmesan cheese.

Kale Salad

Total Prep & Cooking Time: 10 minutes
Yields: 10 Servings

What to Use

- Pepper (as desired)
- Salt (as desired)
- Cranberries (1.25 c dried)
- Sunflower seeds (1.25 c)
- Tomato (2.5 diced)
- Kale (2.5 bunches chopped)
- White sugar (2.5 tsp.)
- Olive oil (2 T + 1.5 tsp.)
- Canola oil (2 T + 1.5 tsp.)
- Lemon juice (1.25 c)

What to Do

- In a serving bowl, whisk together the oil, salt, pepper and lemon juice and combine thoroughly.
- Mix in the cranberries, sunflower seeds, tomato and kale and toss to combine prior to serving.

Watermelon salad with spinach

Total Prep & Cooking Time: 20 minutes
Yields: 10 Servings

What to Use

- Pepper (as desired)
- Salt (as desired)
- Watermelon chunks (5 c)
- Feta cheese (1.25 c)
- Grape tomatoes (2.5 c halved)
- Red onion (2.5 c sliced thin)
- Baby spinach leaves (5 c)
- Arugula (5 c)
- Balsamic vinegar (1T + 2 tsp.)
- Extra virgin olive oil (.3 c + 2 T)

What to Do

- In a serving bowl, whisk together the oil, salt, pepper and balsamic vinegar and combine thoroughly.
- Mix in the tomatoes, onions, spinach and arugula and toss to combine prior to serving. Top with feta cheese and watermelon and serve.

Green Salad

Total Prep & Cooking Time: 10 minutes
Yields: 10 Servings

What to Use

- Pepper (as desired)
- Salt (as desired)
- Feta cheese (5 oz. crumbled)
- Almonds (1.25 c sliced)
- Mixed salad greens (10 c)
- Avocados (2.5 cubed, pitted, peeled)
- Garlic (5 cloves chopped)
- Lemon juice (2.5 tsp.)
- Parsley (2.5 tsp. chopped)
- White sugar (2 pinches)
- Dijon mustard (2 T + 1.5 tsp.)
- White wine vinegar (.25 c + 1 T)
- Olive oil (.5 c + 2 T)

What to Do

- In a serving bowl, whisk together the oil, vinegar, garlic, lemon juice, parsley, sugar, pepper, salt and mustard and combine thoroughly.
- Mix in the salad greens and toss to combine prior to serving. Top with feta cheese and sliced almonds and serve.

Salad with cranberry vinaigrette

Total Prep & Cooking Time: 20 minutes
Yields: 10 Servings

What to Use

- Pepper (as desired)
- Salt (as desired)
- Mixed greens (1.25 lbs.)
- Blue cheese (5 oz. crumbled)
- Red onion (.5 sliced thin)
- Water (2 T + 1.5 tsp.)
- Garlic (.5 tsp. minced)
- Dijon mustard (1 T + .75 tsp.)
- Cranberries (.25 c + 1 T)
- Olive oil (.3 c + 1 T + 1 tsp.)
- Red wine vinegar (3 T + 2.25 tsp.)
- Almonds (1.25 c sliced)

What to Do

- Ensure your oven is heated to 375 degrees F.
- Place the almonds on a baking sheet in a single layer and place the baking sheet in the oven for 5 minutes.
- Add the water, pepper, salt, garlic, mustard, cranberries, oil and vinegar to a food processor and process well.
- Add the blue cheese, onion, almonds and salad greens into a serving bowl, top with the dressing and toss well prior to serving.

Italian salad

Total Prep & Cooking Time: 15 minutes
Yields: 10 Servings

What to Use

- Pepper (as desired)
- Salt (as desired)
- Lemon juice (3 T + 1 tsp.)
- Balsamic vinegar (.3 c + 1 T + 1 tsp.)
- Basil (3 T + 1 tsp.)
- Grapeseed oil (.3 c + 1 T + 1 tsp.)
- Cherry tomatoes (20)
- Green bell pepper (1 sliced)
- Red bell pepper (1 sliced)
- Green onions (.3 c + 1 T + 1 tsp. chopped)
- Red leaf lettuce (1.6 c)
- Radicchio (1.6 c)
- Escarole (1.6 c)
- Romaine lettuce (3.3 c torn)

What to Do

- In a serving bowl, add in the cherry tomatoes, green pepper, red pepper, red-leaf, scallions, radicchio, escarole and romaine lettuce and combine thoroughly.
- In a separate small bowl whisk in the pepper, salt, lemon juice, vinegar, basil and oil and combine thoroughly.
- Combine the two bowls and toss to and serve.

House Salad

Total Prep & Cooking Time: 15 minutes
Yields: 10 Servings

What to Use

- Pepper (as desired)
- Salt (as desired)
- Parmesan cheese (1 c)
- Red wine vinegar (.5 c)
- Extra virgin olive oil (1 c)
- Pimento peppers (4 oz. diced)
- Red onion (1.6 c)
- Artichoke hearts (14 oz. quartered, drained)
- Iceberg lettuce (1.75 heads torn)
- Romaine lettuce (1.75 heads torn)

What to Do

- Mix the pimentos, red onions, artichoke hearts and lettuces together and toss to combine.
- In a small bowl, whisk together the cheese, pepper, salt, red wine vinegar and olive oil. Chill prior to using to top salad. Toss to coat prior to serving.

Chapter 4: Salads for the Entire Family

Sweet potato salad

Total Prep & Cooking Time: 95 minutes
Yields: 4 Servings

What to Use

- Pepper (as desired)
- Salt (as desired)
- Parmigiano-Reggiano cheese (2 in.)
- Baby arugula leaves (.5 lbs.)
- Walnut oil (.5 c)
- Extra virgin olive oil (.5 c)
- Salt (1 tsp.)
- Hot pepper sauce (to taste)
- Dijon mustard (1 tsp.)
- Lemon juice (1 T)
- Shallot (1 chopped)
- Garlic (1 clove minced)
- Red bell peppers (halved)
- Sweet potatoes (4 wedged)
- Olive oil (1 T)

What to Do

- Ensure your oven is heated to 425 degrees F.
- Combine 1 T olive oil with pepper and salt in a small bowl before adding in the sweet potato wedges and tossing to coat.
- Set the bell peppers on a baking sheet and place the sweet potatoes around them.
- Place the baking sheet in the oven for 45 minutes. Shake the pan at the 20 minute mark to prevent sticking.

- Add the shallot and garlic to a food processor and process well, add in the pepper, salt, hot sauce, mustard, lemon juice and peppers and process well. Add in the oils and process well.
- Add the arugula to a bowl and add in the dressing before tossing well.
- Plate the salad, top with potatoes and cheese.

Salad BLT

Total Prep & Cooking Time: 25 minutes
Yields: 6 Servings

What to Use

- Pepper (as desired)
- Salt (as desired)
- Croutons (2 c)
- Tomatoes (2 chopped)
- Romaine lettuce (1 head shredded)
- Garlic powder (1 tsp.)
- Milk (.25 c)
- Mayonnaise (.75 c)
- Bacon (1 lb.)

What to Do

- Add the bacon to a skillet before placing the skillet on the stove over a burner turned to a high/medium heat. Let the bacon cook until crisp and then crumble.
- In a food processor add together the salt, pepper, garlic powder, milk and mayonnaise and process well.

- In a serving bowl, combine the dressing with the croutons, bacon, tomatoes and lettuce and toss to combine prior to serving.

Orzo and spinach salad

Total Prep & Cooking Time: 20 minutes
Yields: 10 Servings

What to Use

- Pepper (as desired)
- Salt (as desired)
- Balsamic vinegar (.5 c)
- Olive oil (.5 c)
- Basil (.5 tsp. dried)
- Pine nuts (.75 c)
- Red onion (.5 chopped fine)
- Feta cheese (.5 lb. crumbled)
- Baby spinach (10 oz. chopped)
- Orzo pasta (16 oz.)

What to Do

- Add the orzo to a pot full of lightly salted water before placing the pot on top of a burner turned to a high heat. Allow the pasta to cook for 8 minutes before draining the pot and running the pasta under cold water.
- In a serving bowl, whisk together the oil, salt, pepper and balsamic vinegar and combine thoroughly.
- Mix in the pasta, pepper, basil, pine nuts, onion and spinach a and toss to combine prior to serving. Top with feta cheese and watermelon and serve.

Asian salad

Total Prep & Cooking Time: 35 minutes
Yields: 6 Servings

What to Use

- Pepper (as desired)
- Salt (as desired)
- Sesame seeds (1 T toasted)
- Green onions (3 chopped)
- Chicken breast (2 halved, shredded, cooked)
- Iceberg lettuce (1 head chopped, dried, rinsed)
- Rice noodles (8 oz. cooked)
- Rice vinegar (3 T)
- Vegetable oil (.25 c)
- Sesame oil (1 T)
- Soy sauce (2 tsp.)
- Brown sugar (2 T)

What to Do

- In a serving bowl, whisk together rice vinegar, salad oil, sesame oil, soy sauce and brown sugar and combine thoroughly. All the dressing to sit 30 minutes prior to serving.
- Add the lettuce, sesame seeds, green onions and chicken to the serving bowl and toss well. Allow everything to chill 10 minutes prior to topping with chicken and serving.

Beet salad

Total Prep & Cooking Time: 40 minutes
Yields: 10 Servings

What to Use

- Pepper (as desired)
- Salt (as desired)
- Goat cheese (2 oz.)
- Extra virgin olive oil (.5 c)
- Balsamic vinegar (.25 c)
- Orange juice concentrate (.5 c frozen)
- Mixed greens (10 oz.)
- Maple syrup (3 T)
- Walnuts (.3 c chopped)
- Beets (4 halved)

What to Do

- Place the beets in a saucepan and cover them with water before placing them on a burner turned to a high heat. Allow them to cook for 20 minutes before draining the water and cubing them.
- Place the walnuts in a skillet and place the skillet on a burner turned to a low/medium heat and allow them to cook until they start to brown before adding in the maple syrup. Coat well and set the walnuts aside.
- In a bowl, whisk together the oil, orange juice and balsamic vinegar and combine thoroughly.
- Add all of the ingredients, save the goat cheese, to a serving bowl and toss well to combine prior to serving. Plate and top with goat cheese.

Avocado salad with strawberries

Total Prep & Cooking Time: 15 minutes
Yields: 2 Servings

What to Use

- Pepper (as desired)
- Salt (as desired)
- Pecans (.5 c)
- Strawberries (10 sliced)
- Avocado (1 sliced, pitted, peeled)
- Salad greens (2 c torn)
- Lemon juice (1 tsp.)
- Apple cider vinegar (1 T)
- Honey (4 tsp.)
- Olive oil (2 T)
- White sugar (2 T)

What to Do

- In a serving bowl, whisk together the oil, sugar, honey, lemon juice and vinegar and combine thoroughly.
- Add the remaining ingredients and toss to coat, chill prior to serving.

Butter lettuce salad with egg

Total Prep & Cooking Time: 55 minutes
Yields: 4 Servings

What to Use

- Pepper (as desired)
- Salt (as desired)
- Chives (.25 c sipped)
- Butter lettuce (1 head)
- Lemon juice (2 T)
- Asparagus (1 lb. chopped)
- Eggs (4 fried)
- Sugar (.25 tsp.)
- Butter (1 stick)
- Sugar snap peas (8 oz.)
- Baby potatoes (1 lb.)

What to Do

- Add the potatoes to a pot and cover them with 2 inches of water before adding a pinch of salt. Place the pot on the stove over a burner turned to a high heat and let it boil before cooking for 10 minutes. Add in the snap peas along with the asparagus and let everything cook about 2 minutes.
- Drain the pot and slice the potatoes.
- Add the butter to a saucepan before placing it over a burner turned to a high heat. Whisk in the sugar, lemon juice, salt and pepper.
- Divide the remaining ingredients between the plates, top with dressing and an egg prior to serving.

Farro salad with cherries

Total Prep & Cooking Time: 30 minutes
Yields: 6 Servings

What to Use

- Black pepper (as desired)
- Sea salt (as desired)
- Parsley (2 T)
- Dried cherries (.75 c)
- Green apple (1 c)
- Basil (.5 tsp dried)
- Oregano (.5 tsp dried)
- Farro (1 c)
- Vegetable broth (2.5 c)
- Walnuts (.25 c)
- Salt (.5 tsp)
- White sugar (2 tsp)
- Apple cider vinegar (.25 c)
- Maple syrup (.25 c)
- Olive oil (.25 c)

What to Do

- In a small bowl, combine the salt, sugar, vinegar, maple syrup and oil and whisk well.
- Add the walnuts to a skillet before adding the pan to a burner turned to a low heat for about 3 minutes until they are well toasted.
- Add the basil, oregano, farro and vegetable broth to a saucepan on top of a burner turned to a high heat. Once it boils, reduce the heat to low/medium and allow everything to simmer about 10 minutes.

- Remove the saucepan from the burner, and let it sit, covered, for approximately 25 minutes to allow the farro to absorb all of the liquid.
- Move the farro to a glass bowl and allow it to cool to room temperature before mixing in the walnuts, parsley, dried cherries and green apples. Mix well and place the bowl, covered, into the refrigerator to chill prior to serving.

Chapter 5: Lunch Salads

Classic Mexican Salad

Total Prep & Cooking Time: 75 minutes
Yields: 8 Servings

What to Use

- Pepper (as desired)
- Salt (as desired)
- Hot pepper sauce (as desired)
- Chili powder (.5 tsp.)
- Cumin (.5 T ground)
- Cilantro (.25 c chopped)
- Garlic (1 clove crushed)
- White sugar (2 T)
- Lemon juice (1 T)
- Lime juice (2 T)
- Red wine vinegar (.5 c)
- Olive oil (.5 c)
- Red onion (1 chopped)
- Corn kernels (10 oz. frozen)
- Red bell pepper (1 chopped)
- Green bell pepper (1 chopped)
- Cannellini beans (15 oz. rinsed, drained)
- Kidney beans (15 oz. rinsed, drained)
- Black beans (15 oz. drained, rinsed)

What to Do

- In a serving bowl, combine the red onion, frozen corn, bell peppers and beans and mix well.

- In a smaller separate bowl combine the pepper, cumin, cilantro, hot pepper sauce, garlic, salt, sugar, lemon juice, lime juice, red wine vinegar and olive oil and whisk well.
- Pour the dressing over the salad and toss well to coat, cover the salad with plastic wrap and allow it to chill in the refrigerator and serve chilled.

Classic Caesar Salad

Total Prep & Cooking Time: 35 minutes
Yields: 6 Servings

What to Use

- Pepper (as desired)
- Salt (as desired)
- Romaine lettuce (1 head torn)
- Bread (4 cups stale, cubed)
- Olive oil (.25 c)
- Lemon juice (1 T)
- Dijon mustard (1 tsp.)
- Worcestershire sauce (1 tsp.)
- Parmesan cheese (6 T grated, divided)
- Anchovy fillets (5 minced)
- Mayonnaise (.75 c)
- Garlic (6 cloves peeled, divided)

What to Do

- Mince the 3 garlic cloves before adding them to a small bowl along with the lemon juice, mustard, Worcestershire sauce, 2 T parmesan cheese, anchovies and mayonnaise and combining thoroughly. Season as desired before refrigerating the dressing.

- Add the oil to a skillet before placing it on a burner turned to a medium heat. Cut the rest of the garlic into quarters and add it to the skillet. Allow it to brown before removing it from the pan and adding in the bread instead. Brown the bread and season as desired.
- Combine all of the ingredients and toss to coat.

Classic black bean salad

Total Prep & Cooking Time: 25 minutes
Yields: 6 Servings

What to Use

- Pepper (as desired)
- Salt (as desired)
- Green onions (6 sliced)
- Tomatoes (2 chopped)
- Red bell pepper (1 chopped)
- Avocado (1 diced, pitted, peeled)
- Corn kernels (1.5 c)
- Black beans (30 oz. drained rinsed)
- Cayenne pepper (as desired)
- Garlic (1 clove minced)
- Olive oil (.5 c)
- Lime juice (.3 c)

What to Do

- Combine the onions, tomatoes, bell pepper, avocado corn and beans in a serving bowl and mix well.
- Add the cayenne pepper, salt, pepper, garlic, olive oil and lime juice to a small jar, cover the jar with a lid and shake well.
- Toss with dressing as desired.

Buttermilk chicken salad

Total Prep & Cooking Time: 30 minutes
Yields: 4 Servings

What to Use

- Pepper (as desired)
- Salt (as desired)
- Romaine lettuce (2 heads torn)
- Olive oil (1 T)
- Chicken breast (24 oz.)
- Parmesan cheese (.25 c)
- Lemon juice (2 T)
- Radicchio (.5 sliced thin)
- Mayonnaise (.25 c)
- Multigrain bread (2 slices)
- Garlic clove (1 pressed)
- Buttermilk (1.5 c)

What to Do

- Mix together the parmesan cheese, garlic, lemon juice and buttermilk and combine thoroughly before seasoning with salt and pepper as desired.
- Add all of the results, expect for .5 c, to a large Ziploc bag before adding in the chicken and shaking to coat. Allow the chicken to sit for up to 24 hours.
- Place the chicken on a foil-lined baking sheet and broil it for 14 minutes or until it reaches an internal temperature of 165 degrees F.
- Combine all of the ingredients in a serving bowl, top with the remaining buttermilk and toss to combine.

Taco salad

Total Prep & Cooking Time: 30 minutes
Yields: 6 Servings

What to Use

- Pepper (as desired)
- Salt (as desired)
- Cherry tomatoes (1 c halved)
- Boston lettuce (2 heads, leaves separated)
- Green salsa (1.5 c)
- Zucchini (1 diced)
- Onion (1 diced)
- White cheddar cheese (1 c shredded)
- Tortilla chips (1.5 c crushed)
- Red bell pepper (1 diced)
- Turkey (1 lb. ground)
- Olive oil (4 T)

What to Do

- Add 2 T oil to a skillet before placing it on the stove over a burner turned to a high/medium heat. Add in the onion and allow it to cook for about 5 minutes before mixing in the turkey and allowing it to cook about 5 minutes.
- Mix in 1 c salsa, red bell pepper and zucchini and cook another 5 minutes, season as desired and remove the skillet from the stove.
- Combine the remaining ingredients in a serving bowl and mix well before plating. Top with the turkey and then the cheese prior to serving.

Spinach salad and poppy dressing

Total Prep & Cooking Time: 15 minutes
Yields: 10 Servings

What to Use

- Pepper (as desired)
- Salt (as desired)
- Almonds (1.25 c slivered)
- Red onion (.75 c + 1 T + 1 tsp. sliced thin)
- Mandarin oranges (10 oz. drained)
- Salad greens (10 c)
- Baby spinach (10 c)
- Poppy seeds (2.5 tsp.)
- White sugar (.75 c + 1 T + 1 tsp.)
- White vinegar (.75 c + 1 T + 1 tsp.)
- Miracle Whip (1.25 c)

What to Do

- In a serving bowl, whisk together the salt, pepper, vinegar, poppy seeds, sugar and Miracle Whip and combine thoroughly.
- Mix in the almonds, onion, oranges, salad greens and spinach leaves and combine well. Toss to combine prior to serving.

Pomegranate and pear salad

Total Prep & Cooking Time: 12 minutes
Yields: 10 Servings

What to Use

- Pepper (as desired)
- Salt (as desired)
- Honey (2 T)
- Dijon mustard (1.5 T)
- Lemon juice (.25 c)
- Pomegranate juice (1.6 c)
- Vegetable oil (.25 c)
- Pomegranate seeds (1.6 c)
- Anjou pear (5)
- Green leaf lettuce (15 c)

What to Do

- Split the lettuce into 10 bowls, divide the pear slices and the pomegranate seeds between them and mix well.
- Separately whisk together the oil, salt, pepper, honey, mustard, pomegranate juice and lemon juice in a saucepan before placing the pan on a burner turned to a high heat. Once it boils, reduce the heat and allow it to simmer, stir regularly until the sauce thickens. Pour dressing over salad and serve.

Conclusion

Congratulations! And thank for making it through to the end of this book, let's hope it was informative and able to provide you with all of the tools you need to achieve your goals whatever they may be.

** Remember to use your link to claim your 3 FREE Cookbooks on Health, Fitness & Dieting Instantly

https://bit.ly/2MkqTit

THE COMPLETE PLANT-BASED COOKBOOK

Introduction

Congratulations on purchasing your copy of *The Complete Plant-Based Cookbook*. I am delighted that you have chosen to take the path of bettering your health through plant-based cooking. Plant-based cooking is a nutritional avenue that allows you to appreciate food in its uncultivated, raw form. The goal of this cookbook is to introduce you to delicious plant-based recipes that are as satisfying as the not-so-healthy comfort foods we have all become so easily addicted to. As daunting as this new cooking lifestyle may be, you will find that these mouth-watering recipes will soon become the new favorite staples in your household.

In Chapter 1, you will notice that the main dishes will require a few more steps to prepare. However, each recipe will provide you with an estimated preparation and cooking time. You will also see the number of servings each recipe can yield, along with its nutritional values, which include the net carbohydrates, protein, fats, and calories. The guesswork has been eliminated for your convenience—unless you want to get creative and add some extra ingredients of your own! The remainder of the book is chock-full of easy-to-follow recipes that will require very little work for highly delicious outcomes.

There are plenty of books on plant-based cooking out there, so thanks again for choosing this one! Every effort was made to ensure that it is full of as much useful information as possible. As always, before implementing any major diet change such as this one, please consult a physician and ensure any questions concerning your nutritional health are answered.

Chapter 1: Main Dishes

Portobello Bruschetta

10 Min. to Get Ready | 5 Min. to Cook
Produces: 4 Servings
Nutritional Score: Calories: 284 | Net Carbs: 13.3 g | Fat: 25.7 g | Protein: 5.4 g

Ingredients:

- ½ C. olive oil
- 6 chopped tomatoes
- 1 C. chopped basil
- 12 cloves minced garlic
- 4 portobello mushrooms
- Salt and pepper

Technique:

- Take 2 T. of oil and 4 cloves of minced garlic to coat each mushroom. Cook in a grilling pan for 5 minutes on each side.
- Mix up tomatoes, basil, remaining garlic, and oil. Fill each mushroom. Top with salt and pepper.

Baked Vegetable Foil Packs

20 Min. to Get Ready | 20 Min. to Cook
Produces: 4 Servings
Nutritional Score: Calories: 97 | Net Carbs: 8 g | Fat: 7.3 g | Protein: 2.3 g

Ingredients:

- 1 peeled and chopped onion
- 1 cut-up yellow squash
- 1 sliced zucchini
- 2 T. olive oil
- Spices of choice

Technique:

- In a bowl, mix all ingredients with olive oil; add spices of choice and toss together.
- Wrap ingredients in foil; make 4 individual packets.
- Cook at 350°F for 20 minutes.

Sweet Potato and Black Bean Tacos

15 Min. to Get Ready | 20 Min. to Cook
Produces: 4 Servings
Nutritional Score: Calories: 430 | Net Carbs: 60 g | Fat: 16 g | Protein: 12 g

Ingredients:

- 4 C. sweet potatoes – no skin, cut in 1" squares
- 1 C. black beans – canned or cooked
- 1 chopped onion
- 2 T. olive oil
- 8 corn tortillas
- 3 minced garlic cloves
- Cilantro

Technique :

- Heat olive oil and add in sweet potatoes. Cook for about 5-6 minutes. Periodically stir.
- Add in onion, garlic, and black beans, cover and let cook for another 10-15 minutes, or until sweet potatoes are at desired readiness.
- Serve in warmed corn tortillas; top with cilantro.

Avocado and White Bean Sandwich

5 Min. to Get Ready | 5 Min. to Cook
Produces: 3 Servings
Nutritional Score: Calories: 325 | Net Carbs: 44.5 g | Fat: 13.1 g | Protein: 9.8 g

Ingredients:

- 1 avocado
- 1 15-oz. can clean white beans
- Juice from 1 lemon
- 1 T. Dijon mustard
- Optional: greens and cherry tomatoes
- Salt and pepper

Technique :

- Drain and clean beans.
- Mash avocado and beans together; add in the rest of the ingredients.
- Spoon onto romaine leaves or gluten-free whole wheat bread.

Veggie-Loaded Rice Bowls

20 Min. to Get Ready | 30 Min. to Cook
Produces: 4 Servings
Nutritional Score: Calories: 547 | Net Carbs: 106.4 g | Fat: 2.1 g | Protein: 26.6 g

Ingredients:

- ½ C. chopped cilantro
- 1 C. pinto beans
- 1 C. black beans
- 1 C. cooked brown rice
- 3 C. spinach
- 1 cut-up zucchini
- 1 chopped bell pepper
- 1 chopped onion
- 1 lime
- 1 t. cumin
- 1 t. turmeric

Technique:

1. Sauté onion and bell pepper for 5 minutes. Add beans and zucchini; cook until warm. Put in your spinach and heat until wilted.
2. Add in cooked rice and spices; stir to combine.
3. Add some juice from a squeezed lime once finished.

Hummus Vegetable Wrap

10 Min. to Get Ready | 25 Min. to Cook
Produces: 4 Servings
Nutritional Score: Calories: 441 | Net Carbs: 68.1 g | Fat: 15.2 g | Protein: 11.7 g

Ingredients:

- 4 whole wheat tortillas
- 1/2 C. hummus
- 4 C. spinach
- 1 cut-up avocado
- ½ thinly sliced cucumber
- 1 thinly sliced bell pepper
- 2-3 shredded carrots
- 1 can cleaned black beans
- 1 C. cooked brown rice

Technique:

1. Warm up your tortillas.
2. On each tortilla, spread a couple of tablespoons of hummus.
3. Top with your cooked rice and the remaining vegetables.

Zucchini Noodle Pasta with Avocado Pesto

15 Min. to Get Ready | 15 Min. to Cook
Produces: 8 Servings
Nutritional Score: Calories: 214 | Net Carbs: 13.2 g | Fat: 17.1 g | Protein: 4.8 g

Ingredients:

- 6 spiralized zucchinis
- 1 T. cold-pressed oil of choice

Avocado Pesto:

- 3 garlic cloves
- 2 cubed avocados
- 1 C. fresh basil leaves
- ¼ C. fresh parsley leaves
- ¼ C. pine nuts
- 3 T. cold-pressed oil of choice
- Juice from 1 lemon
- Salt and pepper

Technique:

1. Spiralize your zucchini and set aside on paper towels.
2. In a food processor, add in all the ingredients for the avocado pesto except the oil. Pulse on low until desired consistency is reached.
3. Slowly add in oil until it's creamy and emulsified.
4. Heat 1 T. of oil and allow your zucchini noodles to cook for 4 minutes.
5. Take your zucchini noodles and coat them with avocado pesto.

Turmeric Roasted Potatoes and Asparagus

10 Min. to Get Ready | 40 Min. to Cook
Produces: 4 Servings
Nutritional Score: Calories: 210 | Net Carbs: 26.4 g | Fat: 11.1 g | Protein: 4.3 g

Ingredients:

- 1l chopped onion
- 1 lb. small red potatoes
- 1 bunch quartered asparagus
- 4 minced garlic cloves
- 2 T. turmeric
- Salt and pepper
- Cold-pressed oil

Technique:

1. Set your oven's temperature to 375°F to preheat.
2. In a dish that's oven-safe, toss the cut-up potatoes with 1 T. of oil and roast for 20 minutes.
3. In another bowl, add asparagus, onions, garlic cloves, turmeric, salt, and pepper. Toss with 1 T. of oil. Add to roasting dish with potatoes.
4. Until potatoes are tender, allow it to cook; it should take around 20 minutes.

Vegan Zucchini Boats

15 Min. to Get Ready | 40 Min. to Cook
Produces: 4 Servings
Nutritional Score: Calories: 228 | Net Carbs: 35.2 g | Fat: 7.4 g | Protein: 8.5 g

Ingredients:

- 2 zucchinis
- 1 C. (2 med. ears) fresh corn kernels
- 1 chopped onion
- 1 can cleaned black beans
- 1 diced bell pepper
- 2 minced cloves of garlic
- 1 diced tomato
- 1 small batch chopped fresh cilantro
- ½ C. quinoa
- 1 ¼ C. vegetable stock
- 2 t.:
    - Ground cumin
    - Chili powder
    - Dried oregano
- 2 T. cold-pressed olive oil

Technique:

1. Set your oven's temperature to 425°F to preheat.
2. Slice both zucchinis lengthwise down the center and carve out the inside to form the "boats." Save the insides for later. Drizzle the zucchinis with olive oil until they're lightly coated; add a sprinkle of salt and pepper. Position the zucchinis

facing down over the prepared baking sheet; place in the oven and cook for around 10-15 minutes.
3. Cook the quinoa in the vegetable stock.
4. In a skillet, stir-fry the onion with 1 T. of olive oil.
5. Add in the remaining vegetables and spices.
6. Add the quinoa to the vegetable mixture; remove from heat.
7. "Stuff" each zucchini boat and place in the oven until tops are browned, which will take about 5-10 minutes.

Tomato Basil Soup

15 Min. to Get Ready | 15 Min. to Cook
Produces: 4 Servings
Nutritional Score: Calories: 53 | Net Carbs: 11.6 g | Fat: 0.5 g | Protein: 2.3 g

Ingredients:

- 1 handful fresh basil leaves
- 3 minced garlic cloves
- 2 15-oz. cans tomatoes – no skin and seeded
- 1 chopped onion
- Salt and pepper

Technique:

1. Sauté garlic and onions for 5 minutes; add in tomatoes.
2. Heat everything thoroughly; remove from heat once you see steam.
3. Add basil, salt, and pepper; transfer to a blender and blend until a soup-like consistency has been achieved.

Thai Peanut Tofu with Sautéed Vegetables

15 Min. to Get Ready | 40 Min. to Cook
Produces: 2 Servings
Nutritional Score: Calories: 834 | Net Carbs: 95.7 g | Fat: 42.3 g | Protein: 24.8 g

Ingredients:

- 1 package pressed and rinsed extra firm tofu
- 1 sliced red onion
- 1 C. packed spinach
- 1 C. shredded carrots
- 1 chopped bell pepper
- 1-inch minced ginger
- 1 small head broccoli – chopped into florets
- 2 minced garlic cloves
- 1 C. quinoa
- 1 can coconut milk
- 2 T. soy sauce
- 1 T. red curry paste
- 1 T. rice vinegar
- 1 T. peanut butter
- 1 t. agave

Technique:

1. Preheat your oven to 400°F.
2. Bake tofu for 20 minutes.
3. Cook quinoa.
4. Sauté garlic, onions, carrots, broccoli, and red pepper for about 5 minutes.

5. Mix in the coconut milk, ginger, soy sauce, curry paste, peanut butter, agave, and rice vinegar. Cook for 5 more minutes.
6. Add the spinach and baked tofu and cook uncovered for 10 minutes.
7. Serve on a bed of quinoa.

Stuffed Peppers

10 Min. to Get Ready | 30 Min. to Cook
Produces: 4 Servings
Nutritional Score: Calories: 668 | Net Carbs: 123.1 g | Fat: 6.1 g | Protein: 34.4 g

Ingredients:

- 1½ C. cooked quinoa
- 1 C. cooked corn
- 4 bell peppers
- 1 15-oz. can black beans

Technique:

1. Preheat oven to 350°F.
2. Combine quinoa, black beans, and corn.
3. Cut off the top and deseed each pepper, then "stuff" and place in a baking dish to cook for 30 minutes.

Chapter 2: Desserts

Dark Chocolate Covered Bananas

10 Min. to Get Ready | 35 Min. to Cook
Produces: 14 Servings
Nutritional Score: Calories: 176 | Net Carbs: 26.6 g | Fat: 8.8 g | Protein: 2.5 g

Ingredients:

- 2 C. dark chocolate chips
- 7 bananas – ripe, cut in half
- ¼ C. almond butter
- 2 T. coconut oil
- 14 popsicle sticks
- Toppings of choice

Technique:

1. Insert a popsicle stick in each banana half, about midway through. Line a cooking sheet with parchment paper for the bananas.
2. Melt the coconut oil in a pan; add in the dark chocolate chips, stir until completely melted.
3. Dip each banana in chocolate, making sure to cover it in chocolate entirely. Place bananas on parchment paper.
4. Drizzle the bananas with almond butter, sprinkle with coconut, cashews, pistachios, or dried cherries.
5. Freeze for 35 minutes.

No-Bake Peanut Butter Cookies Drizzled with Dark Chocolate

15 Min. to Get Ready | 20 Min. to Cook
Produces: 4 Servings (12 cookies)
Nutritional Score: Calories: 235 | Net Carbs: 22 g | Fat: 16.3 g | Protein: 6 g

Ingredients:

- ½ C. dark chocolate chips
- ½ C. peanut butter
- 1 t. pure vanilla extract
- 2 t. coconut oil
- 1 C. dates
- 1 C. almond meal

Technique:

1. In a blender or food processor, add in peanut butter, almond meal, dates, and vanilla extract. Pulse until a smooth consistency is reached.
2. Form dough into 1-inch sized balls and place on a parchment paper-lined cooking sheet.
3. With a fork, press down and make a crisscross pattern.
4. Melt together coconut oil and the dark chocolate chips. Drizzle each cookie with chocolate.
5. Place in the fridge until firm.

Vegan Pineapple Ice Cream

10 Min. to Get Ready | 3 Hr. Freeze Time
Produces: 4 Servings
Nutritional Score: Calories: 460 | Net Carbs: 56.9 g | Fat: 8.2 g | Protein: 41.1 g

Ingredients:

- 1 C. Greek yogurt
- 3 C. frozen pineapple chunks

Technique:

1. Add Greek yogurt and pineapple chunks to a blender and run until smooth.
2. In a freezer-safe container, store until it's frozen.

Matcha & Coconut Power Bars

20 Min. to Get Ready | 45 Min. Freeze Time
Produces: 8 Bars
Nutritional Score: Calories: 430 | Net Carbs: 57.3 g | Fat: 20.9 g | Protein: 11 g

Ingredients:

- 1 T. matcha powder + more for sprinkling
- 2 T. cacao nibs – unsweetened
- ½ C. raw almonds
- ½ C. pecans
- ¼ C. coconut flakes – unsweetened
- 1 ¼ C. pitted and roughly chopped dates
- 1/3 C. hemp seeds
- 1 t. agave

Technique:

1. In a food processor, combine 2 t. of matcha powder, agave, hemp seeds, pecans, almonds, and dates. Pulse until well-combined. The mixture should stick together like dough. If not, add more dates until it does.
2. Add cacao nibs until dispersed.
3. Line a baking sheet with parchment paper. Use hands to press mixture down until smooth.
4. Sprinkle with coconut flakes and extra matcha powder.
5. Freeze for 45 minutes.

Cashew Whipped Cream with Berries

15 Min. to Get Ready | 1 Hr. Cook Time
Produces: 4 Servings
Nutritional Score: Calories: 103 | Net Carbs: 22.1 g | Fat: 3.9 g | Protein: 2.1 g

Ingredients:

- 1 C. raw, unsalted cashews soaked in water for 3 hours
- 1 T. pure vanilla extract
- 2 T. agave nectar
- 2 ½ C. water
- 1 C.:
    - Fresh strawberries – sliced
    - Fresh raspberries
    - Fresh blueberries

Technique:

1. Place soaked cashews in a high-power blender, along with ½ C. water, vanilla, and agave.
2. Blend on high for 2 minutes. Chill for at least 1 hour. This will also help stiffen the whipped cream.
3. Serve on top of fresh berries.

Vegan Dark Chocolate Mint Mousse

10 Min. to Get Ready | 4 Hr. Chill Time
Produces: 2 Servings
Nutritional Score: Calories: 662 | Net Carbs: 56.8 g | Fat: 58.9 g | Protein: 17.1 g

Ingredients:

- 1½ C. coconut milk
- ¼ t. peppermint extract
- 6 T. unsweetened cacao powder
- 4 T. dark chocolate chips for garnish
- 1 T. maple syrup

Technique:

1. Whisk together all ingredients until little air bubbles start to appear.
2. Pour into 2 ramekins.
3. Place in fridge until set; allow up to 4 hours.
4. Top with dark chocolate chips before serving.

Raw Chocolate Brownies

20 Min. to Get Ready | 15 Min. Cook Time
Produces: 2 Servings
Nutritional Score: Calories: 175 | Net Carbs: 33.4 g | Fat: 5 g | Protein: 2 g

Ingredients:

- ½ C. walnuts
- ½ C. almonds
- ¼ C. unsweetened cacao powder
- 1 C. dates
- 2 T. maple syrup

Technique:

1. Soak dates in water for about 10 minutes.
2. In a food processor, pulse nuts until a crumb-like consistency is attained.
3. Remove dates from water, drain, and wring out any excess water.
4. Add the dates, cacao powder, and maple syrup into the food processor. Blend until a smooth but thick consistency is reached.
5. On a piece of parchment paper, roll out brownie mixture into a rectangle, about 1 inch thick. Fold up in parchment paper and chill for 15 minutes.

Banana Almond Chia Pudding

10 Min. to Get Ready | 10 Min. to Cook
Produces: 3 Servings
Nutritional Score: Calories: 299 | Net Carbs: 21.6 g | Fat: 23.6 g | Protein: 4.9 g

Ingredients:

- ¼ C. chia seeds
- 1 C. coconut milk
- 1 C. cashew milk
- 3 T. sliced almonds
- 3 bananas
- 1 t. ground cinnamon
- 2 T. maple syrup

Technique:

1. Whisk together cinnamon, maple syrup, and coconut milk until smooth. Add in chia seeds and let sit overnight.
2. Serve in cold dishes, each topped with one cut up banana and some sliced almonds.

Chocolate Chip Energy Bits

15 Min. to Get Ready | 4 Hr. Chill Time
Produces: 12 Bits
Nutritional Score: Calories: 100 | Net Carbs: 18.2 g | Fat: 2.2 g | Protein: 2.7 g

Ingredients:

- ¼ C. maple syrup
- ¼ C. almond butter
- 1/3 C. mini dark chocolate chips
- 1 C. cooked quinoa
- 1 C. gluten-free oats
- ½ t. vanilla extract
- 1 t. cinnamon

Technique:

1. Knead all ingredients until a sticky dough forms and roll into small balls.
2. Place energy bits on a parchment-lined cookie sheet and refrigerate for 4 hours before serving.

Almond Butter Apple Slices

10 Min. to Get Ready | 5 Min. to Cook
Produces: 4 Servings
Nutritional Score: Calories: 114 | Net Carbs: 19.3 g | Fat: 4.7 g | Protein: 1.7 g

Ingredients:

- 2 apples
- 2 T. dark chocolate chips
- ½ C. almond butter
- 2 T. slivered almonds
- 2 T. shredded coconut – unsweetened

Technique:

1. Remove the core of the apples and slice into rings.
2. Spread almond butter over one side and top with chocolate chips, slivered almonds, and coconut.

No-Bake Chocolate Cookie Dough Bars

15 Min. to Get Ready | 50 Min. Chill Time
Produces: 12 Servings
Nutritional Score: Calories: 341 | Net Carbs: 22 g | Fat: 27.1 g | Protein: 6.1 g

Ingredients:

- ¾ C. dark chocolate chips
- 1 ½ C. almond flour
- 1 t. vanilla extract
- ½ C. maple syrup
- 5 T. nut butter of choice
- 2 ½ T. melted coconut oil

For the Chocolate Topping:

- ½ T. coconut oil
- 2 T. nut butter
- 1 C. dark chocolate chips

Technique:

1. Mix all listed bar ingredients.
2. In an 8-inch baking dish, firmly press dough evenly and place in the freezer for 30 minutes.
3. Melt all chocolate topping ingredients together, pour over the cookie dough bars, and place in the freezer for another 20 minutes.

Triple Berry Ice Cream

5 Min. to Get Ready | 3+ Hr. Chill Time
Produces: 6 Servings
Nutritional Score: Calories: 284 | Net Carbs: 25.2 g | Fat: 17.5 g | Protein: 3 g

Ingredients:

- 1 C.:
    - Raspberries
    - Strawberries
    - Blueberries
- 3 ripe bananas
- 1 15-oz. can coconut milk

Technique:

1. Blend all ingredients.
2. Transfer to a freezer-safe container, cover, and freeze for 3 hours.

Ginger Cookies with Cashew Vanilla Icing

15 Min. to Get Ready | 20 Min. to Cook
Produces: 16 cookies
Nutritional Score: Calories: 197 | Net Carbs: 17.9 g | Fat: 12.6 g | Protein: 4.1 g

Ingredients:

- 1 ½ C. ground oats
- 3 mashed bananas
- ¼ t. sea salt
- 1 T. cinnamon
- 2 T. ground ginger

Cashew Vanilla Icing:

- 2 T. maple syrup
- 1 C. raw cashews – previously soaked for 3 hours
- 2 T. coconut oil
- 2 t. vanilla extract
- Water for blending

Technique:

1. Mix all dry ingredients together; add in the banana.
2. Spoon onto the cookie sheet and bake at 350°F for about 10-15 minutes. You will start to smell the banana when they are done.
3. Make the cashew vanilla icing by adding all ingredients to a blender. Place in the freezer to firm.
4. Let cookies cool completely before putting the icing.

Chapter 3: Smoothies

Blueberry Almond Smoothie

5 Min. to Get Ready | 5 Min. to Make
Produces: 2 Servings
Nutritional Score: Calories: 449 | Net Carbs: 38.7 g | Fat: 33 g | Protein: 8.2 g

Ingredients:

- 1 ½ T. almond butter
- ¾ C. coconut milk
- ½ C. frozen blueberries
- 1 ½ ripe bananas
- 1 T. chia seed

Technique:

1. Using a high-speed blender, process all the listed ingredients until the consistency becomes smooth.
2. If the smoothie is too thick, add more milk until it thins out.

Green Mango Protein Smoothie

5 Min. to Get Ready | 5 Min. to Make
Produces: 2 Servings
Nutritional Score: Calories: 634 | Net Carbs: 56 g | Fat: 47.2 g | Protein: 8.6 g

Ingredients:

- 1 C. spinach
- 2 apples
- 2 C. chopped mango
- ½-inch peeled fresh ginger
- 1 ½ C. almond milk
- 1 T. hemp seed

Technique:

1. Blend all the listed ingredients. Add some ice if you would like to make it colder.
2. If the smoothie is too thick, add more almond milk.

Strawberry Banana Smoothie

5 Min. to Get Ready | 5 Min. to Make
Produces: 2 Servings
Nutritional Score: Calories: 114 | Net Carbs: 26.6 g | Fat: 1.2 g | Protein: 2 g

Ingredients:

- 1 ripe banana
- 2 C. fresh strawberries
- ½ C. dairy-free milk of choice
- Ice – if desired

Technique:

1. Blend all the ingredients together.

Hemp Oatmeal Chocolate Smoothie

5 Min. to Get Ready | 5 Min. to Make
Produces: 2 Servings
Nutritional Score: Calories: 415 | Net Carbs: 56 g | Fat: 23 g | Protein: 20.2 g

Ingredients:

- 1 ripe banana
- 4 T. cacao powder – unsweetened
- 2 T. maple syrup
- 1 C. coconut milk
- ½ C. water
- 4 T. hemp seeds – shelled
- 1 T. oats

Technique:

1. Blend all ingredients on high setting until a smooth consistency is reached.
2. Add more milk if the smoothie is too thick.
3. Add ice if you would like to make it colder.

Vanilla Cashew Smoothie

5 Min. to Get Ready | 5 Min. to Make
Produces: 1 Serving
Nutritional Score: Calories: 569 | Net Carbs: 68 g | Fat: 30.3 g | Protein: 13 g

Ingredients:

- 1/3 C. raw cashews
- 1 banana
- 1 T. chia seeds
- 1 T. maple syrup
- 1 t. vanilla extract OR 1 vanilla bean
- 1/3 C. water
- 1 C. ice

Technique:

1. Blend all ingredients until smooth.
2. Add more water if needed.

Lavender Blueberry Smoothie

5 Min. to Get Ready | 5 Min. to Make
Produces: 2 Servings
Nutritional Score: Calories: 479 | Net Carbs: 34.4 g | Fat: 39 g | Protein: 5.2 g

Ingredients:

- ½ C. ice
- ½ C. chard
- 1 C. fresh blueberries
- 1 C. unsweetened coconut milk
- ½ avocado
- ½ banana
- 1 T. culinary lavender
- 1 t. pure vanilla extract

Technique:

1. Blend everything until smooth and creamy.

Avocado Kale & Raspberry Smoothie

5 Min. to Get Ready | 5 Min. to Make
Produces: 2 Servings
Nutritional Score: Calories: 627 | Net Carbs: 47 g | Fat: 49 g | Protein: 10.4 g

Ingredients:

- 1 handful of kale
- ½ avocado
- 1 C. almond milk
- 1 C. raspberries
- 1 banana
- 1 T. maple syrup
- 2 T. nut butter
- 1 T. flax seed

Technique:

1. Run all ingredients on the blender's high setting until the consistency is smooth.
2. Add ice if you would like to make the smoothie colder.

Tropical Acai Smoothie

5 Min. to Get Ready | 5 Min. to Make
Produces: 1 Serving
Nutritional Score: Calories: 584 | Net Carbs: 77.4 g | Fat: 33 g | Protein: 6.2 g

Ingredients:

- 1 packet acai puree
- 1 banana
- ¾ C. blueberries
- ½ mango
- ½ C. coconut milk
- ½ C. water

Technique:

1. Blend everything together and enjoy!

Green Avocado Smoothie

5 Min. to Get Ready | 5 Min. to Make
Produces: 2 Servings
Nutritional Score: Calories: 369 | Net Carbs: 18.7 g | Fat: 33.9 g | Protein: 3.3 g

Ingredients:

- 1 avocado
- 1 tbsp. maple syrup
- ½ C. almond milk

Technique:

1. Blend all ingredients together.
2. Add more milk if the smoothie is too thick.

Superfood Smoothie

5 Min. to Get Ready | 5 Min. to Make
Produces: 2 Servings
Nutritional Score: Calories: 333 | Net Carbs: 30.8 g | Fat: 24.7 g | Protein: 4 g

Ingredients:

- ¼ C. cucumber
- ½ avocado
- 1 C. spinach
- 1 kiwi
- 1 green apple
- 1 celery stalk
- 2 sprigs mint
- ½ C. coconut milk
- ½ C. water
- Handful of ice

Technique:

1. Blend everything on high; add more water if necessary.

Energizing Kale Smoothie

5 Min. to Get Ready | 5 Min. to Make

Produces: 2 Servings

Nutritional Score: Calories: 190 | Net Carbs: 34.7 g | Fat: 5 g | Protein: 4.5 g

Ingredients:

- 1 ¼ C. fresh kale
- 1 peeled carrot
- 1 banana
- ½ green apple
- 1 T. chia seeds
- ½ C. cashew milk
- ½ C. water

Technique:

1. Blend everything; add more ice if necessary.

Refreshing Pineapple Protein Smoothie

5 Min. to Get Ready | 5 Min. to Make
Produces: 2 Servings
Nutritional Score: Calories: 550 | Net Carbs: 56 g | Fat: 34.2 g | Protein: 14 g

Ingredients:

- 1 C. spinach
- 1 C. fresh pineapple
- 1 kiwi
- 1 C. fresh mango
- 1 orange
- 1/4 C. raw cashews
- 2 T. hemp seed
- 1 T. chia seed
- ½ C. coconut milk

Technique:

1. Blend everything; add water if the smoothie is too thick.
2. Add ice if you would like to make it colder.

Purple Antioxidant Smoothie

5 Min. to Get Ready | 5 Min. to Make
Produces: 2 Servings
Nutritional Score: Calories: 372 | Net Carbs: 46.1 g | Fat: 20.6 g | Protein: 5.7 g

Ingredients:

- 1 C. mixed berries
- 1 packet acai puree
- 1 banana
- 1 beet
- 3 seeded dates
- ½ C. almond milk
- 1 T. chia seeds
- ½ C. water

Technique:

1. Blend all ingredients on high until smooth.
2. Add more water to thin out the smoothie if needed.
3. Add ice if needed.

Chapter 4: Salads

Berry Quinoa Salad

15 Min. to Get Ready | 25 Min. to Make
Produces: 6 Servings
Nutritional Score: Calories: 446 | Net Carbs: 38.9 g | Fat: 28.5 g | Protein: 14.7 g

Ingredients:

- 1 C. cooked quinoa
- 2 C. blueberries
- 2 C. strawberries
- 6 C. spinach
- 2 cubed avocados
- 1 T. hemp seed – per bowl
- ½ C. walnuts
- 2 T. Dijon mustard
- 1 lemon

Technique:

1. In each bowl, start with a bed of spinach; add on a scoop of quinoa, berries, avocado, a sprinkle of hemp seeds, and toss on a few walnuts.
2. Combine Dijon mustard and lemon juice to make the dressing.
3. Drizzle the dressing on top of each salad.

Mandarin Kale Salad with Sweet Tahini Dressing

10 Min. to Get Ready | 15 Min. to Make
Produces: 3 Servings
Nutritional Score: Calories: 550 | Net Carbs: 38 g | Fat: 43.6 g | Protein: 11 g

Ingredients:

- 3 mandarin oranges
- 1 bunch roughly chopped kale
- ½ C. dried cranberries
- ½ C. pecans

Dressing:

- Juice from 1 large orange
- 2 T. tahini
- 1 T. sesame oil
- ½ T. apple cider vinegar

Technique:

1. Combine all ingredients for the dressing and set aside.
2. Prepare each salad by starting with a bed of kale.
3. Each salad will get 1 mandarin.
4. Sprinkle the salads with dried cranberries and pecans.
5. Drizzle with dressing.

Thai Zucchini Noodle Salad

15 Min. to Get Ready | 15 Min. to Make
Produces: 2 Servings
Nutritional Score: Calories: 355 | Net Carbs: 43 g | Fat: 17 g | Protein: 20 g

Ingredients:

- 3 shredded carrots
- 2 spiralized zucchinis – drained of water
- 2 thinly sliced bell peppers
- 10 oz. sliced mushrooms
- 2 t. minced garlic
- ¼ C. peanut butter
- 2 t. freshly grated ginger
- 3 T. liquid aminos
- 1 t. sriracha
- 1 t. maple syrup

Technique:

1. Combine zucchini and carrots; set aside.
2. Make Thai dressing by combining peanut butter, liquid aminos, sriracha, maple syrup, ginger, and garlic together. Whisk well to combine. Add a little hot water to smooth out the dressing.
3. Sauté peppers and mushrooms for about 5 minutes and set aside.
4. Toss all ingredients together; top with dressing.

Tomato Avocado Onion Salad

10 Min. to Get Ready | 10 Min. to Make
Produces: 2 Servings
Nutritional Score: Calories: 613 | Net Carbs: 37 g | Fat: 54 g | Protein: 8 g

Ingredients:

- 2 diced avocados
- ½ sliced red onion
- 1 lb. cherry tomatoes
- 1 cucumber
- ¼ C. chopped fresh cilantro
- Juice from 1 lemon
- 2 T. cold-pressed olive oil
- Salt and pepper

Technique:

1. In a prepared bowl, throw together all the ingredients and drizzle with lemon juice and oil.

Watermelon & Jasmine Rice Salad

15 Min. to Get Ready | 25 Min. to Make
Produces: 2 Servings
Nutritional Score: Calories: 555 | Net Carbs: 99.9 g | Fat: 14.6 g | Protein: 8.3 g

Ingredients:

- ½ C. coconut milk
- 1 C. cut up watermelon
- ½ C. fresh blueberries
- ½ C. chopped fresh basil
- 1 C. cooked jasmine rice
- 2 T. maple syrup
- 1 C. spinach

Technique:

1. Cook jasmine rice according to package directions. Once the rice has cooled, stir in coconut milk and maple syrup.
2. Chop watermelon and basil. Set aside.
3. Lay down a bed of spinach and spoon rice into bowls; add in watermelon, basil, and blueberries.

Mango Black Bean Salad

10 Min. to Get Ready | 10 Min. to Make
Produces: 3 Servings
Nutritional Score: Calories: 669 | Net Carbs: 136.9 g | Fat: 2.8 g | Protein: 33.4 g

Ingredients:

- 2 peeled and diced mangoes
- 3 peeled mandarins
- 1 diced bell pepper
- 1 bunch thinly sliced green onions
- 1 seeded and finely diced jalapeno
- ½ C. chopped fresh cilantro
- 1 C. cleaned black beans
- 1 C. cleaned white beans
- 2 C. arugula
- Juice from 1 lemon
- Juice from 1 orange

Technique:

1. Combine all ingredients together. Each bowl will get 1 tangerine.
2. Squeeze juice from the lemon and orange over the salad.

Red Apple & Kale Salad

10 Min. to Get Ready | 10 Min. to Make
Produces: 5 Servings
Nutritional Score: Calories: 261 | Net Carbs: 26.6 g | Fat: 17.8 g | Protein: 4 g

Ingredients:

- 3 thinly sliced apples
- 2 chopped bunches kale
- ½ C. slivered almonds
- ½ C. coconut flakes

Lemon Dressing:

- Juice from 1 lemon
- 1 minced garlic clove
- 1 t. Dijon mustard
- ¼ C. cold-pressed oil of choice
- Salt and pepper

Technique:

1. Make the lemon dressing by combining all ingredients and whisking until smooth. Set aside.
2. Prepare all salad ingredients; top with dressing and toss to combine.

Cauliflower & Chickpea Salad

15 Min. to Get Ready | 10 Min. to Make
Produces: 4 Servings
Nutritional Score: Calories: 704 | Net Carbs: 89.5 g | Fat: 32.6 g | Protein: 23.4 g

Ingredients:

- 1 head cauliflower – cut into florets
- 1 thinly sliced apple
- 2 cut and cubed avocados
- 1 t. chili powder
- 1 thinly sliced shallot
- 1 handful chopped cilantro
- 1 handful chopped mint
- 1 14-oz. can clean chickpeas
- Salt and pepper

Technique:

1. In your food processor, pulse the cauliflower until its consistency has become rice-like.
2. Toss all ingredients together with a little olive oil and fresh lime juice.

Strawberry Mango and Pineapple Tacos

15 Min. to Get Ready | 5 Min. to Make
Produces: 2 Servings
Nutritional Score: Calories: 452 | Net Carbs: 68.6 g | Fat: 21.6 g | Protein: 8 g

Ingredients:

- 1 C. sliced strawberries
- 1 C. freshly cut up pineapple
- 1 cubed mango
- 1 C. cherry tomatoes
- 1 avocado
- Romaine lettuce leaves
- ¼ C. chopped and soaked red onion
- 1 handful chopped cilantro
- 1 small handful chopped basil
- Juice from 1 lime
- Salt and pepper

Technique:

1. Place romaine leaves on a serving platter.
2. In a small bowl, combine strawberries, pineapple, mango, tomatoes, and herbs. Set aside.
3. In another bowl, mash avocado with onion, lime juice, salt, and pepper. Keep the avocado chunky.
4. Spread a spoonful of the avocado mix on each romaine leaf.
5. Top with fruit mix.

Rainbow Beet Salad

10 Min. to Get Ready | 15 Min. to Make
Produces: 3 Servings
Nutritional Score: Calories: 615 | Net Carbs: 46.8 g | Fat: 44.5 g | Protein: 18.3 g

Ingredients:

- 1 C. spinach
- 1 C. cooked edamame
- 1 cubed avocado
- 1 sliced beet
- 1 sliced bell pepper
- 1 peeled and grated carrot
- 1 C. arugula
- 1 C. fresh blueberries
- ½ C. slivered almonds

Technique:

1. To make the dressing, combine all ingredients and place in the fridge to keep cool.
2. Toast almonds on the stove top until browned.
3. Combine all salad ingredients and top with freshly squeezed lemon juice.

Walnut & Pear Salad with Lemon Poppy Seed Dressing

15 Min. to Get Ready | 10 Min. to Make
Produces: 4 Servings
Nutritional Score: Calories: 408 | Net Carbs: 32.6 g | Fat: 30 g | Protein: 10.1 g

Ingredients:

- 2 sliced pears
- 4 C. spinach
- 1 cubed avocado
- ½ C. dried cranberries
- 1 C. walnuts

Lemon Poppy Seed Dressing:

- 3 T. avocado oil
- 3 T. cold water
- 1 t. Dijon mustard
- ½ t. onion powder
- ¼ t. lemon zest
- Juice from 2 lemons
- 1 T. poppy seeds
- 1 T. maple syrup
- ¼ t. sea salt

Technique:

1. Whisk together all the dressing ingredients and chill until salad is ready.
2. Toss all the salad ingredients together and top with dressing.

White Bean & Asparagus Salad

10 Min. to Get Ready | 15 Min. to Make
Produces: 2 Servings
Nutritional Score: Calories: 600 | Net Carbs: 50.2 g | Fat: 39.6 g | Protein: 18 g

Ingredients:

- ½ C. cleaned white beans
- ½ pound cut and blanched asparagus
- 1 cubed avocado
- 1 chopped bell pepper
- ¼ C. chopped parsley
- 1 t. dried oregano
- 2 C. arugula

Dressing:

- ½ T. cold-pressed olive oil
- 1 T. fresh lemon juice
- 1 T. Dijon mustard
- Salt and pepper

Technique:

1. Combine all ingredients for the dressing and store in the fridge until ready to use.
2. Blanch the asparagus by boiling for 3-5 minutes until tender. Run under cold water once done.
3. Toss all the salad ingredients together and serve on top of the arugula.
4. Drizzle with dressing.

3 Bean Salad with Roasted Sweet Potatoes

20 Min. to Get Ready | 30 Min. to Make

Produces: 2 Servings

Nutritional Score: Calories: 906 | Net Carbs: 135 g | Fat: 30.8 g | Protein: 30.4 g

Ingredients:

- 1/3 C.:
    - White beans
    - Pinto beans
    - Black beans
- 1-pound peeled and diced sweet potatoes
- 1 diced red onion
- ½ C. cilantro
- 1 minced garlic clove
- ¼ C. pumpkin seeds
- Juice from 1 lime
- 1 t. chili powder
- ¼ t. sea salt
- Cold-pressed oil

Technique:

1. Preheat your oven to 400°F.
2. Toss sweet potatoes and onions with 1 T. of oil. Bake until sweet potatoes are at the desired tenderness. This will take about 35 minutes.
3. Mix together lime juice, garlic clove, chili powder, sea salt, and 1 T. of oil to make the dressing.
4. Rinse and drain the beans.

5. Once the sweet potatoes and onions are done, transfer to a large bowl. Combine with beans, cilantro, and pumpkin seeds.
6. Drizzle with dressing.

Conclusion

I hope you enjoyed your copy of *The Complete Plant-Based Cookbook*. Let's hope it was informative and that it provided you with a good foundation of recipes that will allow you to easily live the plant-based diet lifestyle.

** Remember to use your link to claim your 3 FREE Cookbooks on Health, Fitness & Dieting Instantly

https://bit.ly/2MkqTit

Binge Eating

Binge Eating Guide to Stop and Overcome Overeating

Introduction

Congratulations on purchasing the *Binge Eating: Guide to Stop and Overcome Overeating* and thank you for doing so. Obesity is omnipresent today. In many cities over half of the adults are obese, and many of the children are as well. One of the largest contributors to obesity is binge eating. Binge eating is when someone is driven to eat compulsively and keeps eating passed the point of fullness and even passed the point of physical pain. It is often done in an altered state of consciousness in which the eater doesn't even notice what she/he is eating. Binge eating, quite often, is a contributing factor to the diabetes epidemic.

The following chapters will discuss the causes of binge eating and learn how to stop it. By learning what triggers a binge eating episode, a person is empowered to break the cycle that keeps them unhealthy and unhappy. Also explained is why diets will not make you thinner nor stop overeating. The bad habits that keep you locked into continuing binge eating are described along with an easy way to do away with them. A guide to making a food plan that will give you complete control over your food intake is included. Finally, a chapter devoted to strategies for continued success in avoiding binge eating and its associated maladies.

There are plenty of books on this subject on the market, thanks again for choosing this one! Every effort was made to ensure it is full of as much useful information as possible, please enjoy!

Chapter 1: Identifying and Overcoming Causes of Bingeing

You tell yourself you aren't going to give in this time. You just need to be a little bit stronger. It's just a question of will power. You hold out for a while, and then give in to the urge to binge. Cookies, ice cream, fried rice, tacos- it doesn't matter. Even though it is food that you love, you don't particularly enjoy it. You mindlessly eat it. Maybe all at once or maybe you pick at it all day. You might not even remember eating it afterward. Finally, you start to feel sick and over full. But you keep eating. Just a little more... and then you can't eat anymore. There is physically no room left in your stomach. Unable to eat anymore, all that is left is to get rid of the evidence and begin the self loathing and shame cycle. This is what it is like to be binge eating.

Bingeing is compulsive behavior. It is ritualized and patterned. It is driven by the subconscious. You have little control over it. The urge to binge can be all consuming. It doesn't begin and end with over eating. It is a cycle, a system that perpetuates itself. There is a trigger, an eating session, and then shame and feeling sick. These after effects leave you more susceptible to starting the cycle over again and again.

There are serious repercussions to binge eating. Obesity and diabetes are most often associated with bingeing. Each comes with potentially overwhelming health and monetary costs. There are long term mental health complications that arise from binge eating also. Negative body image and shame associated with eating disorders can spur depression and feelings of helplessness. Aside from the serious long term effects, there are immediate effects too. Nausea, abdominal pain, and low energy have an impact on quality of life, as does the ill feeling that comes from putting your body through a binge.

The cause of binge eating is not known. It is likely a combination of psychological, environmental, and biological factors- all acting on the subconscious mind. The act of bingeing is done in an altered state of consciousness. Because these are both areas largely out of our conscious control, the best way to fix the problem is to deal with something we have some control over: triggers.

Anything can serve as a trigger. There are probably as many triggers as there are people. It just depends on the individual what will or will not spur them to binge. It could be smell, a thought, stress at work or home, or even just a bad habit.

Recognizing your triggers is necessary to interrupt the cycle and stop binge eating.

Some triggers are easily recognizable. The most obvious is hunger. It is the most obvious, and the hardest to overcome in the moment. The hungrier you are the more food you will make/order, and the more you will eat. In fact, being hungry all but guarantees that you turn your next meal into a session of overeating followed by feeling ill and being ashamed.

Not all triggers are obvious. Many are hidden within our psyches and even into our metabolic function. Meaning your body is triggering itself to overeat and binge. Dehydration can be a trigger. Sometimes the body sends a message to consume water by making you thirsty. But because all food contains some water, the body can also signal you to eat to replenish water stores.

Low levels of necessary nutrients in the system my lead to binge eating, as the body calls for more food replace them. Whatever the trigger, knowing about them is the first step in dealing with them.

Not getting enough sleep can make you less alert and therefore more susceptible to over eating. When you don't feel well you can make poor decisions and get caught in a bingeing cycle. By itself, lack of sleep can cause weight gain. Add in binge eating and you can see how sleep deprivation rally works against you in your pursuit of better health.

Many triggers may be hard to avoid, like stress. You never know when you will have trouble at work or with a spouse. The world is a stressful place and random undesirable things happen. How do you avoid the unavoidable? You don't. There are a variety of stress reducing things you can do to calm yourself. Meditation, exercise, breathing exercises, or some other method may be used to keep you from overeating.

Mental health can also trigger over eating. Depression and other mental health issues can cause us to binge eat. Food can be used to self medicate. It soothes and elates us the same way that drugs do. It makes sense that we would try to alleviate the anguish of mental illness with food leading to the need for help from mental health care professionals.

The single best way to end the urge to binge is to recognize the triggers and traps that lead us into bingeing and other undesirable behavior. Knowing what your triggers are gives you the first bit of control over binge eating. Putting that knowledge to work is the next step in the battle. Practice walking away from triggers that apply to you. Make not getting caught in these traps a habit. The more you do it the easier it becomes. Keeping yourself fed and hydrated. Choosing higher quality fresh foods whenever possible to maximize health and well being is the key to sustaining a binge free life. Take care of yourself and make an effort to stay fit and active. Be sure to get enough sleep. Sleep deprivation can spur weight gain and declining health, which put you at increased risk from triggers. With enough self care, unhealthy eating habits and their effects can be minimized.

Chapter 2: Manage your food

We eat food in order to make energy for ourselves to do all the things necessary to survival and to replenish the raw materials needed to build and repair the tissues of the body. Unfortunately, many of the foods we eat today are very high in calories, and very low in nutrients. This has led to a population that is both obese and malnourished! In addition to obesity, the food we eat is causing diabetes, and general poor health. For the binge eater, the effects of this diet are multiplied.

The foods consumed during binge eating tend to be almost exclusively the worst parts of an already unhealthy diet. Bingeing on the extremely high calorie foods like processed sweets, fatty meats, and fried foods can add a full days worth of calories in only a few minutes. Eating these sugary processed foods can be catastrophic to a person's health. It gets worse. There are at least three ways in which processed foods can *cause* or, at least facilitate, binge eating.

Blood Sugar Spike

Foods that are high in refined sugar as well as simple carbohydrates (bleached flour products) are very easily metabolized by the digestive system. They can be broken down into glucose (blood sugar) in just a few minutes. Glucose is the fuel we use to power our bodies systems. The levels of glucose in our blood spikes when we eat sugars and simple carbohydrates because the body breaks them down into fuel which is deposited into the bloodstream very quickly. In other words, we get a big shot of fuel available to us... too much, in fact, to use all at once. The body reacts to high blood sugar by releasing insulin, which starts the process of storing that excess energy as fat. As the glucose levels go down, so does our energy. This cycle of extremely high blood sugar followed by extremely low blood sugar is what causes diabetes. It can also trigger and eating binge. When our blood sugar gets really low, eating again brings it back up. The body sends signals that compel us to eat, and overeating is often the result. This is a feedback loop of cause and effect that is very easy to get caught in, and can be difficult to get out of.

Quality foods like fresh fruits and vegetables, lean meats, and fish, are harder for the body to break down and extract energy from. The result is slower rise in blood sugar without the unhealthy spike. The sugars extracted from good food slowly trickle into the blood stream and provide consistent energy for hours, rather than minutes. Think of it as the difference between throwing a log on a fire and throwing a can of gas on a fire. The gas will release huge amounts of energy, but it will all be gone in a few seconds. The log will continue to burn and provide heat for a long time.

Processed Foods are Nutrient Poor

Another aspect of the fast food/boxed food diet is that is generally low in nutrients necessary to good health. Processing foods, such as milling, boiling, and preserving, strips away valuable vitamins, minerals, and other nutrients. Our bodies react to the lack of nutrients by insisting we eat more in order to recoup them. Another self perpetuating cycle- the foods we eat don't nourish us and our bodies demand more of them, even when we are not hungry, in a vain attempt to replenish nutrient stores. Many processed foods contain chemical additives which are not digestible. In order to get rid of these chemicals, the body depletes itself further of necessary nutrients to eliminate the additives.

Nutrient rich foods replace the stores of vitamins and minerals the body needs. This is why eating a healthy quality meal satisfies without necessarily feeling full. The body was lacking in nutrients, not calories.

Sugar is Addictive

Probably the most insidious aspect to a diet high in sugar is that it can be highly addictive. More and more, scientists are coming around to the evidence that sugar can be as addictive as hard drugs such as cocaine. Sugar, in high doses, alters brain chemistry the same way that cocaine and heroin do. Like other addictive drugs, the more sugar is ingested, the more you want to eat. It is yet another cyclical pattern that reinforces itself in the binge eater.

Limiting or avoiding processed sugar is the best way to deal with the addiction. But more important that removing foods from your diet is adding in as much nutrient dense food as your body needs to grow, heal, and power itself. Foods like lean meats, fresh fruits and vegetables, fish, nuts, and seeds will give you all the building blocks and consistent energy you need. It's not a question of choosing good food over bad food. If you eat good foods that you like and that are healthy, you will likely find that you want less of the processed food.

Deciding when to eat can be as important as what to eat. Meals should be spaced out to minimize hunger. Hunger is the worst trigger of all for binge eating. If you are ravenously hungry, there is very little possibility of avoiding an eating binge. An ideal schedule would have breakfast served as late in the morning as possible- but not so late that hunger pangs cause you to over eat. The later that breakfast is eaten, the longer the "fasting period" between dinner the night before and breakfast. The longer the fasting period is, the more calories are consumed. Similarly, eating dinner earlier will lengthen the fasting period thereby promoting weight loss. Again, dinner shouldn't be so early that you get hungry again before bed, because that will eventually lead to overeating.

Controlling what foods you eat and when you eat them can alleviate many of the factors that lead to binge eating. Switching to a high quality food diet that limits the intake of processed foods will do the most to help you live a healthier life.

Chapter 3: Put an End to Dieting and Other Bad Habits

Fad diets don't work. Most diets will help you lose weight in the short term. But the overwhelming majority of people gain all the lost weight back. Often they gain back more than they lost in the first place. Diets are usual very restrictive in both the types of foods you can eat and in quantity. It can be hard work to stay on a diet. Especially if you don't enjoy the types of foods you are allowed to eat. Diets feel like punishment, and eventually we walk away from them and into the waiting arms of a food binge.

Diets are designed to fail. We think of diets as temporary suffering that we can stop once we lose the weight we want to be rid of. So even if you do manage to lose every ounce of weight you wanted to lose, there is nothing to keep you from gaining it all back once you stop the diet. Few people make it even that far. Diets are usually broken long before weight loss goals are met. Failing at a diet makes us feel weak and hopeless. Dieting is a one of many bad habits that lead to binge eating.

Food addictions, like drug and alcohol addiction, can be very difficult to control. Habits, on the other hand are relatively easy to change. Habits form out of repetition and routine. There is little if any emotional attachment to a habit. Undoing a bad habit can be as simple as doing something else over and over until it becomes habitual. A few common bad habits that feed over eating are:

Waiting Too Long to Eat

You think that if you hold out and wait before eating you will lose more weight. Or maybe you just lost track of time and didn't realize it until you were very hungry. Either way you are now likely to overeat. It is next to impossible to not to when you are a binge eater. This habit is easily broken by planning meal times and having food prepared and ready to go.

Free Day (binge day)

Some people believe that allowing yourself to binge periodically will get the urge out of your system. One day a week you allow yourself to eat whatever you want in whatever quantities. This is a bad idea because it reinforces the idea that binge eating is an acceptable sometimes. Very quickly it will start happening more often and then everyday is potentially a free day.

Eating in the Car

We all do it, but it is a bad habit, especially for binge eaters. In the car you are insulated from the outside world and you can eat in private. This is exactly how many people prefer to binge eat. The types of foods you eat in the car are almost entirely processed packaged or fast food. So even if you don't binge in the car, the foods you eat there are sure to be empty calories at best.

Nothing but Processed Food in the House

Eating only processed foods can cause overeating as discussed in the previous chapter. Having only these types of foods on hand means that is what you will eat when you get hungry. You should always have good foods readily available.

Eating Foods We Do Not Like

We think that in order to lose weight and get healthy, we have to suffer. Part of that suffering is eating foods we don't like because they are good for us. If you get hungry and only have kale in the house to eat, you may well end up going out and getting fast food. Buy and eat healthy foods that you want to eat.

Thinking of Exercise as Punishment

We tend to think of exercise as penance for over eating. When we think of it this way, it is drudgery. You have to force yourself to go, and you can't wait for it to be over. It doesn't take long before you stop going entirely. Exercise, like healthy foods, must be enjoyable for there to be any chance of you sticking with them. Choose something you enjoy doing for exercise. Being active is one of the best things you can do for yourself. Find something you like and do it.

Snacking

Snacking can be an effective way to curb your appetite or hold you over until the next meal. More often than not, however, it is just a bad habit that can quickly devolve into binge eating. If you must have snacks, limit them to healthy foods in small portions.

Alcohol

Drinking alcohol lowers inhibitions and often ends in overeating. An alcohol fueled binge is particularly bad because there are a lot of calories in most forms alcoholic beverages. A night of drinking can mean consuming as many calories as a whole meal. Heavy drinking can cause you to take in more calories than you should in a full day worth of meals. Drinking less often and eating a good meal before drinking can help, but avoiding it as much as possible is best.

Giving up dieting is easy. Changing other bad habits is generally fairly easy also. A little planning ahead solves most of them the rest just need a good habit to replace them. The benefit from giving them all up is much improved ability to avoid bingeing episodes.

Dieting does not help. Many of us have been on diets our whole lives. We don't permanently lose weight on diets, and worse they keep us in a cycle of starving ourselves, then bingeing, then feeling ashamed and back to dieting. It is a trap that holds us back from doing the work that will actually heal us. Other bad habits have a similar effect. Eliminating bad food related habits clears the road of obstacles to better health. It is the start if building a plan for how you will eat going forward.

Chapter 4: Create Sustainable Eating and Living Habits

As we have seen, diets will not help you lose weight. They won't help you with binge eating either; in fact dieting can be part of the cycle that leads us into binge eating. When a diet fails us, we go into chaotic and unplanned eating. These are the times when we do the most damage to ourselves with food. Food choices are made in the moment and tend to be processed comfort foods. We crave the foods we were prohibited from eating in diet we just quit. Even if it doesn't taste good, we eat it in rebellion against the oppression of the diet. Chaotic eating isn't a solution, so what should we do? The answer is to be smart about how you eat. Choose good foods and plan meals in advance.

Diets fail because they are restrictive and take your favorite foods from you. Instead of taking foods away, add in high quality nutrient dense fresh foods. Eat enough of these foods to energize and satiate your body.

It is important to remember to find the healthy foods that you like to eat. Everyone likes the idea of kale, but nobody actually likes to eat kale. If you try to force yourself to eat it, you are tempting a backlash binge. Eating food should be pleasurable, not tedious. If you enjoy eating this way you will continue doing it. If not you won't. You are not limited to just healthy foods. Other less healthy foods can still be eaten, but they are no longer the focus of the meal. Since you can eat what you truly want, there is no restriction to rebel against. If you crave something you can have it, just make sure you take care of all your bodies nutritional needs first.

Planning your meals gives you ultimate control over your food intake. When you decide what you are going to eat ahead of time, you can choose foods that replenish and nourish you. You have more control over portion size when you pre plan a meal. Most people eat whatever is in front of them even if it is more than they really wanted. By setting a portion size before hand, you can reduce over eating. You can also control the amounts of processed foods you eat. This allows you to have the foods you crave but in smaller quantities mixed with nutritious foods.

Having a meal plan also includes deciding when to eat. As discussed previously, the timing of meals plays a role in avoiding triggers, as well as maximizing the use of the energy derived from the food. Spacing meals farther apart increases the number of calories burned, but also runs the risk of increased hunger and increased risk of binge eating. Finding a balance between the two is necessary and dependent on your goals. If weight loss is the primary reason for changing your eating habits, then spread out you meals more, especially the time between dinner and breakfast. If ending binge eating is your primary concern, shortening the time between meals would be better.

An important decision to make in your food plan is whether or not you want to allow snacking. Snacks can be trouble. When we binge eat, we don't consciously think about the food or eating it. In other words we are not mindful of our food. When you eat something you enjoy, the food should have your full attention. If you are mindlessly eating it and not even noticing it, why bother eating it at all? Snacking is usually not mindful eating. We eat something while we are working or watching television. This may be why snacking leads us into overeating so easily. But if you plan snacks, they are ok. Pre-portioned high quality and tasty snacks can hold you over between meals and keep you from getting to the ravenously hungry point where bingeing is inevitable. By having a food plan, you can make snacking a beneficial part of your daily routing. Without planning, snacking is an invitation to binge.

By planning the foods you eat and scheduling the times you eat them, you eliminate many of the pitfalls that lead to binge eating. You also give yourself the ability control your food intake and tailor it to accomplish the goals that you set. You decide if you want to tailor your plan to lose weight, manage overeating, or both.
Along with a food plan, a plan for getting enough sleep and exercise will make your eating plan much more successful. Sleep and exercise strengthen and replenish you.

Finding a form of exercise that you genuinely enjoy and scheduling yourself time to do it regularly further enhance your ability to control your eating and your life. Ideally you would do something that you like to do and look forward to. If it is something that you want to do, there is a much better chance of you continuing to do it.

Finally, getting enough sleep is necessary to get the full benefits from how you eat and exercise. A full night's sleep will allow you to lose weight. When you are sleep deprived, your body holds on to the weight, and it is extremely difficult to lose it. Exercise breaks down muscle and bone. The body repairs and strengthens muscle and bone best when you sleep. Good food, exercise, and proper sleep will help you look and feel your best. How you see yourself goes a long way toward how you treat yourself.

Now you have the tools to change how you eat and how you feel. You have control over many of triggers that spark binge eating. The effects of triggers not under your control can be muted or avoided entirely because of the plans you have in place. With these tools the drive to binge eat can be severely weakened or done away with entirely. The last part of the puzzle is maintaining the food plan and further insulating you from a possible relapse.

Chapter 5: Self-Acceptance and Avoiding Relapse

Once you have your triggers under control and are eating healthy nourishing meals at regularly scheduled times and all is going well, how do you avoid a relapse? As discussed in earlier chapters, avoiding triggers is extremely important. But sometimes the triggers are difficult to avoid. Having a negative body image makes seeing yourself in the mirror a potential trigger. It's is pretty difficult to avoid yourself, so if negative body image is a trigger for you, then you'll have to find ways to improve how you see yourself.

Negative body image means feeling uncomfortable in your own skin. You don't believe you are attractive or are worthy of attraction from others. You feel anxiety and shame about the size of your body and you see yourself as a failure for allowing it to happen.

It can act as a trigger for some, but even if it doesn't directly lead to over eating and bingeing it can play a role in a relapse. When you feel good about how you look, doing the work to look and feel healthy is easier. If you don't like the way you look, it can drag down your mood and ability to make healthy choices. Maintaining a positive body image of ourselves is important to maintaining a binge free life. If, every time you see yourself in the mirror you get depressed, you may end up in an overeating cycle. This chapter is about improving body image and other ways to reduce the risk of backsliding into overeating.

The causes of negative body image are in large part due to the presentation of ideal bodies as normal in media. Children grow up in a world believing that the flawless bodies they see in media are what they should look like, and that they are flawed. We get caught up comparing ourselves to the perfect bodies we see, and we find ourselves lacking. Feeling this way about your body can make you feel overly self conscious in public. Negative feelings about your appearance are negative feelings about who you see yourself to be. There are ways to combat negative body image.

Accept Yourself for Who You Are

Nobody is perfect. You want to look like that actor or supermodel? It isn't possible. *They* don't even really look like that! Teams of trainers, dieticians, makeup artists, sleep therapists, plastic surgeons, and others are paid a lot of money to keep them looking as good as humanly possible. Even with all that help, and a professional photographer under perfect lighting, their pictures still get photo shopped. Perfection does not exist. These enhanced images of enhanced people are shown to you specifically to make you feel inferior, so that you will buy more products.

Ignore the Media
Avoid media offerings that only feature "ideal" body imagery and discussion. The advertising, fashion, and entertainment industries are not your friend when it comes to body image. Nothing will make you feel bad about your body image faster than comparing yourself to a six foot tall super model with amazing curves and a pencil thin waist, or that perfectly chiseled actor with the 6-pack. It's easy to fall into the trap. Images of perfect bodies are everywhere. But, if you look away from the magazine rack, television, or your phone and look at the people around you. They don't look like the people in those pictures either. They probably look a lot like you.

Focus on Positives

Find a couple of things about your body that you do like and focus on those things when negative thoughts come up. Better yet, try to see yourself through the eyes of someone who adores you. What is it they like about your body? Instead of berating yourself for imperfections focus on your positive qualities. Do the same for other people. There is no good reason to make negative comments about your body or other people's bodies either.

Get Some Exercise

Not only will exercise make you feel better and look better, it can make you feel strong and confident. Like with food choices, choosing a form of exercise you find enjoyable will make it easier to stick with it. Hiking, swimming, paddle boarding, team and individual sports, or anything else that will raise your heart rate and make you sweat a little bit. Ideally, you would find a challenging physical activity that you enjoy to the point that it becomes something you look forward to.

Exercise is very important to staving off binge eating even for those without body image issues. The strength and energy boost that comes with regular physical activity make it easier for you not need to overeat.

Get Some Sleep

Not getting adequate sleep can be damaging to body image. It can make you gain weight and it can make you look older and, well, tired. Sleep is rejuvenating. Your body repairs and restores itself while you sleep. You will look healthier because you'll be healthier. A full night's sleep can also invigorate the spirit as energy levels rise.

Cut Yourself Some Slack

Relapses happen. There is really no point in beating yourself up for falling off the wagon. Getting upset about a relapse puts you back into a shame cycle that got you here in the first place. Recognize that this is a difficult problem, and there will be setbacks, but that you are on a viable path to healthiness and you will succeed. All you can do is give yourself the best chance to succeed every day.

Take Care of Yourself

The way to beat binge eating is through self care. Caring for yourself with good food that satisfies all your body's needs and your need to enjoy what you eat. Getting enough sleep and exercise to make you healthier and happier is self care. Encouraging a positive body image is also caring for yourself by accepting and even liking who you are. So, take care of yourself and stay healthy!

Conclusion

Thank for making it through to the end of *Binge Eating: Guide to Stop and Overcome Overeating*, let's hope it was informative and able to provide you with all of the tools you need to achieve your goals whatever they may be.

The next step is to decide that you want to change your life. Are you ready to do the work necessary to make your life better? To get off the path that leads to obesity, diabetes, poor mental and physical health, and an early death? It starts with the will to change.

Now that you know why some foods and eating habits cause obesity and diabetes, you can make informed decisions on what to eat and how much. Factor in choosing what times you eat, and you have the ability to tailor you food plan to achieve the specific goals you have set. Whether you choose to lose weight, just steer clear of binge eating, or both, is up to you.

It sounds like a lot of work. Fortunately, the steps advocated in this book are relatively easy. You are not asked to give up foods you love or be expected to sweat in misery as you do exercises you hate. You are not asked to diet at all. Actually, you should quit dieting altogether. Dieting will not help you, and in fact it can hurt you, by causing you to rebel and go back to binge eating. Dieting is often part of the cycle of binge eating that is keeping you from living life to the fullest. For these reasons, dieting should be rejected.

Finding ways to heal yourself of bingeing that are sustainable- meaning they are enjoyable to do so it is easier to keep doing them, is the key to lasting life change and freeing yourself from overeating. You can change your life, and you now have the tools to do it.

So go out and live your best life. A life full of fun activity and healthy joyful eating that is worth living. Be free from binges and the shame and self harm that come with them. Enjoy being fully energized and healed by the food you eat, and not dragged down by it. Live in the confidence that you will succeed, even if you have a relapse, the path back to health is here for you. Be comfortable in your body and confident around other people without being victimized by negative body issues. Live as an example to others that binge eating can be conquered.

Fitness Nutrition:

How to Unlock Your Physical Potential by Working Out and Eating Properly

Introduction

Congratulations on purchasing the *Fitness Nutrition* and thank you for doing so.

The following chapters will discuss how to unlock your unlimited potential, look great through healthy eating, and work out according to your physical needs.

There are plenty of books on this subject on the market, thanks again for choosing this one! Every effort was made to ensure it is full of as much useful information as possible, please enjoy!

Imagine your dream body... got it? Alright, now realize you can achieve your dream body through intense workouts and delicious recipes that are simple and easy to follow. Nutrition is the single most important aspect of looking and feeling great.

In this book, there are 11 workouts ranging from cardio to HIIT (High-Intensity Interval Training), to simple bodyweight exercises... to workouts that require zero equipment whatsoever.

EVERY SINGLE WORKOUT can be done at home; you do not need fancy gym equipment to achieve what you desire, all that is needed is the mindset.

The following weight lifting workouts include:

- Chest, shoulders, and triceps
- Back, biceps, and abs
- Upper and lower abs
- Obliques and hips
- Inner and outer thighs

- Hamstrings, quads, and calves
- A total butt workout

Here is the equipment you will need: a yoga mat, weight bench, or a fitness ball, dumbbells, barbells (almost little to no weights are needed), and a medicine ball.

Every exercise includes a warm-up sequence that is necessary to prevent injury and to help you burn more fat. It is important to cool down after every workout. You can go for a five or ten-minute walk around the block or your apartment/house or do some easy yoga positions. The cooldown is entirely up to you. It is recommended that you work out three-days-a-week, targeting different muscles groups for each day, and then give yourself a rest day for proper muscle development. If you follow the routine and recipes I have covered in this book, you are guaranteed excellent results.

Chapter 1:
Chest, Shoulders, and Triceps

It is vital that you warm up the muscle groups that you plan on working on that day. If you do not, there is a serious risk of injury when the muscles and joints are not properly prepared.

Warm-up

1. **March in Place:**
   March in place for 60 seconds. Do your best to not only walk at a fast pace but also lift your knees as high as they will go.

2. **High Knees:**
   This is an exaggerated version of marching in place. This is meant to keep your heart rate elevated and to help you burn more calories. You are going to quickly run in place, keeping your elbows touching your waist with your forearms and palms extended parallel to the floor. Try your best to touch your knees to your palms as quickly as possible for 60 seconds.

3. **Boxing Squat Punch:**
   Place your feet shoulder-width apart while you keep your back straight as you squat. Keep your hands at your chest and stick your butt out when you squat. As you rise, alternatively rotate to your left and right-side punching after you squat. Raise up, punch to the left with your right arm, rotating your right foot into the punch. Drop into a squat, rise, then punch to the right with your left arm. Repeat for 60 seconds.

4. **Big-Arm Circles:**
   Bring your arms up above your head and make a "V." Then make big, wide circles with your arms. Going forward for 30 seconds. Reverse the direction for another 30 seconds.

5. **Wrist circles:**
   Bring your hands together at your breastplate and interlace your fingers. Move only your wrists for 60 seconds.

Workout

1. **Barbell Shoulder Press:**
   Place your feet so they are just outside of the imaginary vertical line you could draw down from your shoulders. With your palms facing inwards, grip the bar, keeping your hands a little wider than your shoulders – make sure your wrists stay straight. Keep your elbows forward a little bit past the barbell, this will help keep the barbell in place. Press the barbell upward and as you are doing this, push your head through your arms once the barbell is above your head. Do four sets of reps; 15-12-10-5

2. **Single-Arm Upright Row:**
   Hold a dumbbell in one hand at your side, palms facing back. Bring the dumbbell up to chin height, keeping your elbow higher than your wrist. Slowly drop the dumbbell back to starting position. Repeat on the other side after one set. Do four sets of reps: 15-12-10-5

3. **Dumbbell Incline press:**
   Put your weight bench on an incline or place your fitness ball against a wall and sit at an angle with a straight back resting

on the ball. Keep your feet and knees wide. Hold in each hand a dumbbell near your shoulders. Press the weights upward while you squeeze your chest muscles. The dumbbells should come closer together naturally when you raise them up, but they do not need to touch, then slowly lower your weights back into the starting position. Do three sets of reps: 15-12-10-5

4. **Bent over Delt Fly:**
Hold a dumbbell in each hand, keep your feet a little wider than your shoulders, and make sure your knees slightly bent. Bend forward at your hips until your chest is just about parallel to the ground. Keep your back completely straight with your palms facing down and then raise the weights out and up to the sides as high as they will go. Keep your movements controlled. Do three sets of reps: 15-12-10-5

5. **Seated Dumbbell Press:**
Sit on a bench holding your dumbbells at chin height with your elbows out to the sides and your palms in a forward facing position. Press the weights fully above your head for a full extension – keeping your shoulders down will help to isolate your triceps and chest. Do three reps of 15.

Chapter 2: Abs, Back, and Biceps

Warm-up

1. **<u>Cat-Cow Stretch:</u>**
   Get on all fours with your hands and knees shoulder and hip length apart. Gently arch your back, rounding up and tuck your chin and tailbone in underneath you. Inhale and as you exhale, drop your back and lift your tailbone like it is being pulled up with a string. Look up towards the sky as if you were trying to make a "U" shape with your back. Repeat 10 times.

2. **<u>Toe Touch:</u>**
   While you are standing, keep your feet together and reach up towards the sky with your hands. Fold forward at the hips and push your hips back as you reach for the floor, shifting your weight on to your heels. Keep your back straight. Then we are going to lift and, to do this properly, we are going to gently round the spine and lift one vertebra at a time, finishing in the starting positions. Repeat 15 times.

3. **<u>Triangle position:</u>**
   While standing, take a big step forward with your right foot into a lunge position. Do not let your knee pass your ankle and maintain a straight left leg by dropping your knee. Since you lunged forward with your right side, you are going to take your left hand and place it on the ground just to the left of your right foot. Take your right arm and reach straight up to the sky and follow your reach with your gaze. You should be making a straight line with both arms. Repeat on the right and left side five times.

4. **Side-Stretch:**
   Place one palm on a wall and bring your entire inner arm to meet the wall as well. Rotate your chest away from the wall and then hold for 20 seconds. Repeat alternatively on each side six times.

5. **Plank:**
   Get into a push-up position with your feet together and your wrists directly beneath your shoulders. Hold for 30 seconds

Workout

1. **Wide-grip pull-ups:**
   Place your hands facing forward and grip a pull up bar slightly wider than your shoulders. Squeeze your core and back to help you lift. Try not to use your shoulders or arms.

2. **Bent Over Rows:**
   Place your feet hip-width apart bending your knees slightly. With weights in each hand, bend forward at your hips and not at the waist. Keep your core engaged and your arms hanging, and your elbows tucked into your sides. With your palms facing each other, squeeze your shoulder blades and bring your elbows up tightly against you as you bring the weights up to your armpits. Imagine you are cracking an egg with your shoulder blades when your elbows are up. Hold for one count and then release. Do three sets of 8-12 reps.

3. **Bent Over Bicep Curls:**
   Begin by doing a bent over row and as you release to go back to the starting position, face your palms towards your chest

and curl your weights to your chest. Engage your biceps at the height of the curl. Do not swing your arms to do this exercise, use only your muscles. Lower your weight amount if you need to. Do three sets of 8-12 reps.

4. **<u>Rear Delt Flies:</u>**
   Start by placing your feet about hip-width apart and bend over slightly at the hips while squeezing your core. Have your arms holding weights slightly in front of your knees. While you bend over slightly, open your arms out to the sides as high as possible, squeezing your shoulder blades together. Do not swing your arms, use your back and core to lift. Slowly release your arms, and do not stop engaging your abs. Do three sets of 8-12 reps.

5. **<u>Basic Crunch:</u>**
   Start out by laying on your back with your feet on the floor, and your knees slightly bent. Press your fingers lightly at the base of your skull to support your head. Engage your core to lift your upper body as much as possible and never stop squeezing your core. Transition into the next exercise after crunching for 15 seconds.

6. **<u>Bicycle Crunches:</u>**
   Remain in the crunch position with your back on the floor. Extend your feet just above the floor, before bringing one of your knees up towards your body and raising your body slightly to touch it with the opposite elbow. Keep your core engaged as you push your foot back and bring the other knee up to touch it with your other elbow. Maintain a lifted upper body and twist for your elbow to meet the opposite knee. Repeat for 15 seconds.

7. **Swimmers:**

    Lay on your stomach with your arms and legs extended. Lift your arms and legs while engaging your core. Drop your left leg and right arm down, then lift those back up as your drop your right leg and left arm down. Alternate sides like you are swimming. Do not completely drop your arms or legs. Repeat for 60 seconds.

8. **Plank:**

    Get into a pushup position with hands and feet shoulder length apart. With your wrists directly underneath your shoulders, engage your core and hold for 30 seconds.

Chapter 3:
Hamstrings, Quads, and Calves

Warm-up

1. **Leg Swings:**
   Begin by standing in an upright position. Take one leg and swing it back and forth. Keep your core engaged while you maintain a straight leg without moving your upper body. Repeat 20 times with each leg. After you complete both legs, switch to a side to side motion with the opposite leg in front of the leg that is stationary. Repeat for 20 seconds on each leg.

2. **Frankenstein Walk:**
   Kick a straight leg out in front of yourself and extend the opposite arm to touch your shin as you slowly walk forward. Repeat 20 rep. Total.

3. **Quad Walk:**
   Stand on one leg while pulling the opposite leg to meet your buttocks and stretch as far as you are able. Alternate each leg 20 times

Workout

1. **Squat with dumbbells:**
   Your feet should be shoulder width apart with your toes pointing slightly outward. Hold your dumbbell at the top like a cup and let the lower part of the weight hang down. Keep your back straight as you lower yourself on to an invisible

chair, making sure you sink into your heels. Once your thighs are parallel, squeeze your glutes, and legs as you lift. Repeat for 45 seconds.

2. **Dumbbell Squats:**
   Stand with your feet about two fist lengths apart, holding dumbbells at your sides. Point your toes slightly outward. Do not lift the weights with your arms. Move into a low squat while keeping your back straight, shifting your weight from your toes to your heels. Keep your chest up as much as possible. Lift back up using only your legs and transition your weight back to your toes with your chest puffed out slightly whilst leaning back. Repeat for 45 seconds.

3. **Lunges:**
   Place a footstool against a wall and place your legs about hip-width apart, keeping your arms at your sides holding weights. Step forward with one foot onto the footstool, causing your thigh and calf to be at a 90-degree angle. Make sure your knee does not go past your ankle. As you drop into the lunge position, your back knee should lower slightly. Push back into starting position. Repeat 6-12 times, then repeat on the opposite leg.

4. **Wall Squats:**
   Hold a medicine ball against a wall with your lower back, with weights in your hands. Stand with your feet about one step out and hip-width apart, making sure your toes are ahead of your knees. With your weights hanging at your sides, roll down the wall until your legs make a 90-degree angle. Squeeze your legs and glutes to raise your body back up, keeping your knees slightly bent. Repeat for 45 seconds.

5. **<u>Deadlifts:</u>**
   Start with your feet slightly wider than your hips and hold a barbell with no weights on top of your thighs (you can always add weight later) with your hands just on the outside of your hips. Lock your legs and *slowly* lower the barbell towards your feet, keeping your back straight. Remember to keep your core flexed, as this protects your back. Keep the barbell close to your legs on your way down. Lift back up with a straight back and make the barbell take the exact path going down. Repeat as many times as you can do in perfect form.

6. **<u>Squat and Hold:</u>**
   Place your back against a wall with your feet about hip-width apart and one step ahead of you. Stack your knees on top of your ankles as you drop into a squat. Make sure your knees are slightly behind your toes. Hold for 60 seconds.

Chapter 4: Cardio HIIT

Warm-up

1. **Shoulder and Head Rolls:**
   Assume the starting position by standing up tall with a straight back. Lift your shoulders and roll them forward to make a circle. That is a shoulder roll. To roll your head, gently tilt your head and neck forward, then rotate 360 degrees gently without forcing your neck. Do 15 reps of each.

2. **Upper Body Twist:**
   Stand with your feet on either side of your body, slightly wider than your hips. Bring both hands up, level with your chest, then make loose fists and rotate your torso and hips to the left along with your hands. Pause and hold for three seconds. Then return to the beginning. Rotate to the left, then repeat eight times.

3. **Hip Circles:**
   Start in a standing position – your feet should be about shoulder-width apart – and rest your hands on your hips. Push your hips to the front then slowly rotate in a clockwise manner. Perform 5-10 rotations then switch the direction.

4. **Knee Circles:**
   Place your feet shoulder-width apart and bend your knees slightly forward. Place your hands on your knees and while you keep your feet on the floor, rotate your knees clockwise. Keep your hip movements to a minimum. Do 5-10 reps in one direction and then switch.

5. **Arm Circles:**
Extend your arms straight out to the sides with your shoulders down. Rotate your arms forward in small circles for five reps. Reverse the direction for five reps. Repeat the whole process in big circles.

6. **Knee Lifts:**
Lift one knee as close to your chest as possible and hold with your hands. Hold this position for three seconds. Lower the foot. Repeat with opposite knee. Do 10 reps.

Workout

1. **180-degree jump squats:**
Start out with your legs slightly wider than your hips and your toes pointed outward. Begin in a low squat position, then jump up and spin 180-degrees, then land softly back in a squat position. Reverse the direction each time. Repeat for 45 seconds.

2. **High Knees:**
Engage your abs while you run in place quickly, lifting your knees as high as you can. Repeat for 45 seconds.

3. **Crazy Jumping Jacks:**
Squeeze your core and extend your arms out to your sides making 90-angles, your fingers pointing up. Lift your left knee out to the side and up, then lower your left elbow to touch your left knee. Simultaneously drop the left knee while you repeat the motion on the other side. Repeat for 45 seconds.

4. **Crisscross Pick-ups:**

Start out with feet shoulder width apart, jump down into a squatting position. As you lightly engage your core, touch the floor with your right hand. Jump up in the air and crisscross your legs, then land back in to squat position. Touch the floor with your left hand. Repeat for 45 seconds.

5. **Butt Kickers:**
Keep your feet shoulder-width apart. Quickly kick your left heel towards your glutes. As you lower your left foot, kick your right leg back at the same time. Repeat for 45 seconds.

6. **Star Jumps:**
Begin by placing your feet roughly shoulder width apart and keeping both your arms close to your body. Squat halfway down reaching your right toes with your left hand. Quickly jump up and spread your arms and legs out like a starfish. Land softly back into a half-squat position, touching your left toes with your right hand. Repeat for 45 seconds.

7. **Plank Jacks:**
Start in a plank position with your wrists under your shoulders and keep your feet together. Engage your core while you hop your feet out wide and then hop back into the starting position. Keep your back straight and your upper body still. Repeat for 45 seconds.

8. **Cross-over punch:**
Start out in a half squatting position with your feet shoulder-width apart. Keep your shoulders relaxed and your core engaged; make fists, then punch to the left with

your right hand. Repeat by punching to the right with your left hand. Repeat for 45 seconds.

Chapter 5: Abs

Warm-up

1. **<u>Bear Crawl:</u>**
   Begin by getting on all fours with both hands directly underneath your shoulders and your knees directly beneath your hips. Using your toes, grip the floor and lift your knees a couple of inches off the floor. Move forward by simultaneously moving your left leg and right hand at the same, then right leg and left hand. Crawl forwards in this manner 10 yards, and then backward 10 yards

2. **<u>Spiderman Planks:</u>**
   Begin in the plank position with your hands underneath your shoulders. Bring your right foot up and plant it outside your right hand. Hold for 15 seconds, keeping your back straight and your front knee directly above your ankle. After that, keep your balance with your left arm, lift your right hand reaching all the way up to the ceiling, following your reach with your gaze. Hold the position for 15 seconds, then return to starting position. Repeat both these stretches on both sides of your body.

3. **<u>Body Saw:</u>**
   Get into a plank position with your feet hip-width apart, then drop your elbows, so they are directly underneath your shoulders. Keep your body and back straight as you rock back and forth, maintaining a tight core. Do 10 reps.

4. **<u>Plank:</u>**
   Get into a traditional plank stance and hold the position for 10 seconds. Do 3 reps of 10.

Workout

1. **Diamond Back:**
   Lay face down on the floor with your glutes squeezed so that your legs lift high off the floor. Engage your core and lift your chest completely off the floor with your arms directly in front of you, pull one elbow into your back, then alternate arms while you keep your chest and legs elevated. Repeat for 60 seconds.

2. **Scissor Clap:**
   Lay on your back while you engage your core and lift your shoulder blades off the floor. Lift your right leg, keep it straight as you clap your hands behind your knee. Keep your back straight, and your core tight along with your shoulder blades lifted as you repeat on the other side. Repeat for 60 seconds.

3. **Low Side-Plank Knee Lift:**
   Begin by getting into a side plank position with your forearm on its side, your elbow directly underneath your shoulder, and your legs extended and straight. Place your feet on top of each other. You want to make a straight line with your body. Lift your top elbow up in the air, then place your hand at chest level with your palm facing your toes. Lift your top knee to tap your palm, then lower back down. Repeat for 60 seconds – 30 seconds on each side.

4. **Ab Sprint:**
   Sit on your bottom with your back straight and one of your legs extended straight out in the air. Your other leg is brought close to your body, so your knee is close to your

torso. Alternate your legs while pumping your arms as if you were sprinting. Repeat for 60 seconds.

5. **Drumming in V:**
Begin on your bottom again with your legs lifted straight at a 30-45-degree angle. Keep your torso lifted and your back straight like you are making a "V" with your body. Engage your core, make fists, then lightly bang on your abdomen like it is a drum, alternating your hands. Repeat for 60 seconds.

6. **Piking:**
Begin in a high plank position with your feet slightly apart. Hop your feet towards your hands and with your back straight, your core tight, and your butt piked towards the ceiling. Hold for one count, then hop back into the plank position for one count. Repeat for sixty seconds.

7. **Alternating planks:**
Begin in a high plank position, then extend your left arm ahead of you and your right leg out behind you, slightly higher than your spine. Hold for one count and then switch the arm and leg. Repeat for 60 seconds.

Chapter 6: Obliques

Warm-up

1. **Bear Crawl:**
   Begin by getting on all fours with both hands directly underneath your shoulders and your knees directly beneath your hips. Using your toes, grip the floor and lift your knees a couple of inches off the floor. Move forward by simultaneously moving your left leg and right hand at the same, then right leg and left hand. Crawl forwards in this manner 10 yards, and then backward 10 yards

2. **Spiderman Planks:**
   Begin in the plank position with your hands underneath your shoulders. Bring your right foot up and plant it outside your right hand. Hold for 15 seconds, keeping your back straight and your front knee directly above your ankle. After that, keep your balance with your left arm, lift your right hand reaching all the way up to the ceiling, following your reach with your gaze. Hold the position for 15 seconds, then return to starting position. Repeat both these stretches on both sides of your body.

3. **Body Saw:**
   Get into a plank position with your feet hip-width apart, then drop your elbows, so they are directly underneath your shoulders. Keep your body and back straight as you rock back and forth, maintaining a tight for. Do 10 reps.

4. **Plank:**
   Get into a traditional plank stance and hold the position for 10 seconds. Do 3 reps of 10.

Workout

1. **Wood Choppers:**
   Stand with feet hip-width apart and hold a dumbbell on its side with both hands diagonally above your right shoulder, placing your weight on your right foot. Twist towards your right hip as you make a chopping motion down past your left hip. Return to your starting position. Do this for 20 reps on each side of your body.

2. **Russian Twist:**
   Sit up high on your butt with your feet flat on the ground and your knees bent. Lean back slightly while you keep your back straight. Using a dumbbell, hold it on the outsides of the weight, cross your ankles, then lift your feet off the ground. Continuously rotate from left to right touching the weight to the ground as you twist from side to side. Repeat for 45 seconds.

3. **Side Plank Lifts:**
   Assume a side plank position. Place your free hand on your hip. Lift your lower body to make a straight line. Lower your hip to the floor and immediately raise it back up for one count. Repeat for 20 seconds on each side.

4. **Bicycle Crunches:**
   Assume the crunch position with your back on the floor. Extend both feet just above the floor, before bringing one of your knees up towards your body and raising your body slightly to touch it with the opposite elbow. Keep your core engaged as you push your foot back and bring the other knee up to touch it with your other elbow. Maintain a lifted upper body and twist for your elbow to meet the opposite elbow. Repeat for 15 seconds.

Chapter 7: Outer and Inner Thighs

Warm-up

1. **Leg Swings:**
   Begin by standing in an upright position. Take one leg and swing it back and forth. Keep your core engaged while you maintain a straight leg without moving your upper body. Repeat 20 times with each leg. After you complete both legs, switch to a side to side motion with the opposite leg in front of the leg that is stationary. Repeat for 20 seconds on each leg.

2. **Frankenstein Walk:**
   Kick a straight leg out in front of yourself and extend the opposite arm to touch your shin as you slowly walk forward. Repeat 20 rep. Total.

3. **Quad Walk:**
   Stand on one leg while pulling the opposite leg to meet your buttocks and stretch as far as you are able. Alternate each leg 20 times

Workout

1. **Thigh burns with wide leg jumps:**
   Put your feet into a wide squat stance. Bring your hands to your heart level and press your palms together. Your hips should be in line with your shoulders. Engage your core then jump up and land in a squat; make sure your knees are above your ankles. Repeat for 45 seconds.

2. **Dumbbell squats:**

Place your feet wider than your hips. Hold a dumbbell in each hand shoulder width apart with your hands facing each other. Your arms should be hanging directly under each shoulder. Engage your core to help keep your back straight and protected. Squat down low while your knees stay above your ankles. Return to the starting position. Do three reps for 30 seconds each.

3. **Plank Lifts:**
Get into a high plank position and lift one leg parallel to the ground and hold for 45 seconds. Complete two reps on both sides.

4. **Stepping Squats:**
Start with your feet hip-width apart. Lower yourself into a half squat then step as far left with your left foot as you can, then bring your right foot in to put yourself back at the starting position. Repeat for 30 seconds on each side.

5. **Outer Leg Lifts:**
Lay on your right side with your right hand supporting your head. Keep your hips stacked on top of each other. Lift your top leg up and pump it up about 10 inches. Do not let your leg drop or bend. Switch sides. Do three reps for 30 seconds.

Chapter 8: Butt

Warm-up

Reference Chapter Three

Workout

1. **Squat Pumps:**
   Stand in a squat position, then drop into a low squat. Begin to pump your butt up and down for 45 seconds

2. **Lunges:**
   Place your hands on your hips while standing up straight. Step forward with one foot about three feet, drop both of your knees and bend them to 90 degrees keeping your shoulders in line with your hips. Repeat for 30 seconds on each side.

3. **Squats:**
   Begin by getting into a wide squat stance then drop into a low squat. Squeeze your glutes on the way up. Repeat for 45 seconds.

4. **Plank kick:**
   Get into a plank position with your knees lowered down towards the floor. Lift one leg up and pump it up as high as you can get it to go. Repeat on each side for 45 seconds.

Chapter 9: Back

Warm-up

Reference Chapter 2.

Workout

1. **Elevated Pushup:**
   Put your hands wide on the floor with both of your feet elevated on a bench or couch. While looking down and keeping your back straight, do a pushup. Do three reps 20 seconds each.

2. **Swimmers:**
   Lay on your stomach with your hands and feet extended. Engage your core, then lift one arm up along with the opposite leg. Drop down and continuously alternate for 45 seconds.

3. **Reverse crunches:**
   Lay on the floor on your stomach, place your hands at the base of your skull while engaging your back muscles. Lift your chest off the floor, then lower back down for one count. Repeat for 45 seconds.

4. **Rear Delt Flies:**
   Start by placing your feet about hip-width apart and bend over slightly at the hips while squeezing your core. Have your arms holding weights slightly in front of your knees. While you bend over slightly, open your arms out to the sides as high as possible, squeezing your shoulder blades together. Do not swing your arms, use your back and core to lift. Slowly

release your arms, and do not stop engaging your abs. Do three sets of 8-12 reps.

Chapter 10:
Nutrition and Fitness go Hand in Hand

Have you ever wondered why working out constantly never seems to give you the results you require? Most likely it is because of your diet. Incorporating the best diet into your life encourages the reduction of body fat, increased energy, extra weight loss, and protection against illnesses. Nutrient dense foods are the most important aspect of fitness. Studies have shown that not eating before you work out will help you to burn 20% more fat than if you ate prior. Eating meals rich in protein after a workout is crucial to the process of repairing and building muscle.

Losing weight is only 20% exercise, the other 80% is dieting. What you eat matters in terms of weight. Reduce your sugar intake by reducing your consumption of sodas and processed sugary treats. Drink plenty of water before, during and after a workout. When you crave something sweet, opt for a piece of fruit. Instead of eating three large meals a day, switch to eating 6 or 7 small meals. To increase your metabolism, it is best to workout right after you wake up, plus you will begin to have more energy during the day. Always eat breakfast – ___always___. This gives you the fuel you need to start the day and keeps you sharp. Incorporate complex carbs along with protein first thing in the morning, this will help regulate your blood sugar and gives you fuel for hours without a crash.

If you are trying to build muscle, you need to eat before and after a workout. Eat carbs with a little protein, and then after working out go protein crazy. For every pound you weigh, you need to consume 0.7 grams of protein every day. Protein is the most readily available nutrient on the planet, and there are countless sources other than meat and dairy: nuts, nut butter, beans, legumes, whole grains, nut milk, yogurt, soy, quinoa, most vegetables. You will also need to limit your saturated and trans fat intake, like candy and fried foods.

Eat healthily and eat often. Drink plenty of water. The reason complex carbs are a great combination is that carbs give your body energy and protein helps to build muscle, skin, and hair. Both are required for a faster metabolism and for building muscle. When you want to lose weight and gain muscle, and/or slim down: pairing the perfect balance of nutrition with cardio, weight-training, and rest days will help you to achieve the perfect body you have always dreamed of.

Chapter 11: Top SEVEN Delicious Plant-based Recipes PACKED with Protein

1. Breakfast Banana Shake

Ingredients:

- Banana (1, frozen and sliced)
- Soy Milk (1 cup, unsweetened)
- Hemp Seeds (2 Tanlespoons)
- Chis Seeds (1 tablespoon)
- Maca Powder (1 Tablespoon)
- Protein Powder(1 scoop, preferably Vegan)
- Peanut Butter (2 Tablespoons)

Preparation:

Place all of the ingredients into a blender and blend on high until the consistency is completely smooth.

2. Tofu Scramble

Ingredients:

- Olive Oil (1 teaspoon, extra virgin)
- Onions(.25 cup, chopped)
- Bell Peppers (1 cup, red and green)
- Spinach (1 cup)
- Tofu (13 ounces)
- Pinch of Salt
- Pinch of Pepper

Preparation:

Heat the olive oil in a pan until hot. Add onions and bell peppers. Sauté until soft and brown. Add Tofu, spinach, salt, and pepper. Sauté for a little while longer on medium heat. Enjoy!

3. Chickpea and Red Pepper Salad

Ingredients:

- chickpeas (2 15-ounce cans, no salt added, drained and rinsed)
- Bell Peppers (3 red, finely diced)
- Cilantro(handful, chopped)
- Parsley(1 cup, chopped)
- Garlic(3 cloves, minced)
- Olive Oil (1 tablespoon, extra virgin)
- Lemon Juice(2 Tablespoons)
- Pinch of salt
- Pinch of pepper
- Whole Wheat Pitas

Preparation:

Toss all the ingredients into a big bowl and refrigerate for at least two hours, letting all the flavors come together. After the mixture is chilled, spoon it into a pita.

4. Southwestern Quinoa Bowl

Ingredients:

- Quinoa(.5 cup, prepared)
- black beans(.5 cup prepared)
- extra firm tofu(6 ounces)
- spinach or kale(2 ounces)
- bell peppers(.5 cup, chopped)
- tomato(1 small, diced)
- cilantro with green onions(.25 cup, chopped)
- Lime juice
- Pinch of Salt
- Pinch of pepper

Preparation:

Add the beans and quinoa, along with vegetables to a bowl. Toss together with salt, pepper, and lime juice.

5. Almond Butter and Banana Sandwich

Ingredients:

- Banana(1 very ripe, sliced)
- Almond Butter(2 tablsepoons)
- chia seeds(1 Tablespoon)
- whole grain bread(2 slices)

Preparation:

Spread almond butter on to bread. Add banana and chia seeds.

6. Almond Butter and Pomegranate Quesadillas

Ingredients:

- Pomegranate Seed(.33 cup)
- Banana(1 large, sliced)
- Almond Butter(e Tablespoons)
- Whole Wheat Tortillas(2 large)
- Cinnamon(.5 teaspoon)

Preparation:

- Preheat a large skillet over medium-high heat. Drizzle with coconut oil.
- Prepare the quesadillas, spread 3 tablespoons of almond butter on each tortilla. Leave 1 inch from the border.
- One Tortilla shell will have the sliced banana, pomegranate seeds, and cinnamon.
- Fold in half.
- Cook in the skillet for approximately 3 minutes, or until each side is brown.

7. Black Bean Enchiladas

Ingredients:

- Tortillas(10-12)
- Cumin(1 teaspoon)
- Cilantro(.5 cup, chopped)
- Green onions(4-5, sliced)
- Corn(1.5 cups, frozen or fresh)
- Black Beans(1 15-ounce can, rinsed and drained)
- Avocados(2 small or medium)
- Quinoa(.5 cup, uncooked)

For the Sauce:

- Vegetable Broth(3 cups)
- Chili Powder(.25 teaspoon)
- Onion powder(.25 teaspoon)
- Garlic powder(.25 teaspoon)
- Paprika(.5 teaspoon)
- Cumin(2 teaspoons)
- Olive oil(2 teablespoon)
- All-purpose Flour(.25 cup)
- Tomato Paste(.25 cup)

Preparation:

- Rinse, then cook qionoa according to directions on the package; using 1 cup of water.
- Make the enchilada sauce: Combine flour and spices. Then warm the olive oil over medium heat in a sauce pan.
- Once heated, add in the tomato paste and the flour and spices combination.

- Cook for 1 minute while whisking. Then add in broth, then boil. Reduce heat to a simmer. Continue to whisk for another minute or two.
- Chop the avocado and green onions.
- In a bowl, combine the beans, onions, corn, cumin. Toss in the cooked quinoa, stir. Then add in the avocado.
- Preheat the oven to 375 defrees Fahrenheit. Lightly coat a baking dish, coat the bottom with a small amount of sauce.
- Distribute the bean mixture to the middle of each tortilla. Roll them up then place the seam side down in the dish.
- Pour the rest of the sauce on top of the unchiladas.
- Bake for 25 mintues

Conclusion

Thank you for making it through to the end of *The Fitness Nutrition*, let's hope it was informative and able to provide you with all the tools you need to achieve your goals, whatever they may be.

The next step is to start working out!

- **** Remember to use your link to claim your 3 FREE Cookbooks on Health, Fitness & Dieting Instantly**
- **https://bit.ly/2Lvj2Pm**

The Complete Bodyweight Training:

How to Use Calisthenics to Become Fitter and Stronger

Introduction

Congratulations on downloading this book and thank you for doing so.

What has been holding you back from achieving your fitness goals? Is it the complication of the various gym equipment? Because gym memberships cost you more than you should be spending (especially if you hardly have any time to hit the gym)? Or is it the lack of proper guidance that assures you that you're on the right track and working your muscles the way you should?

Whatever the reason may be, there is now an answer and a way for you to achieve the physique you have been aspiring to build – through bodyweight training exercises.

Bodyweight training is exactly that –*using your own body to train and get fitter.* Yes, because getting fit doesn't have to involve a lot of complicated machinery or excessive cost. Why, when your body is a powerful machine on its own, that is just waiting to be utilized to the fullest? You don't need various equipment to get the results you want, all you need to do is to be training in the right way and this book – right here – is where you begin to make those changes.

In the following chapters, you will begin to discover just how to effectively increase your total body strength without the need for free weights, fitness machines, or even a gym membership. That's right, all you are going to need is the strength of your own body, determination to stick to these bodyweight training exercises and follow this complete and easy to follow guide to the most effective bodyweight workouts that will make a difference.

Bodyweight training exercises are *the best* thing for your body because it is something everyone at all fitness levels can do. That's because one of the significant benefits of these exercises is that they can be adapted and modified to your body and fitness level, simple yet challenging at the same time.

There are plenty of books on this subject on the market, thanks again for choosing this one! Every effort was made to ensure it is full of as much useful information as possible, please enjoy!

Chapter 1: Why Bodyweight Training Kicks Butt

Have you ever bodyweight trained before? If you haven't, then it's about time that you started.

Why?

Because bodyweight training is going to *kick your butt.* In a good way, of course.

Contrary to popular belief, there is no need to be hitting the gym hard, seven days a week for an hour or more at a time to see visible results. You don't need to be pushing yourself to the point of exhaustion, trying to utilize all those machines, dumbbells and kettle balls to see an actual difference.

Not when all you need is the strength and the power of your own body. Bodyweight training is a key element of fitness building that is very often underutilized because it doesn't seem like it would be effective enough to get the desired results. But that is where you are mistaken because bodyweight training exercises are effective. *Super effective.*

If you need more convincing about why you should begin harnessing the power of bodyweight training, here is a list of what this form of training and exercising can do for you:

- **Cardio and Core All-In-One** – If you're short on time (as a lot of us often are), then bodyweight exercises are going to be the best workouts to squeeze in a calorie-burning session that still packs a powerful punch. Some bodyweight training exercises combine both cardio and strength in one, which keeps your heart pumping, burns the fat while building strength and muscle definition at the same time.

- **Easy Transitions** – Because bodyweight training is going to be using no equipment at all, it will be easy to transition quickly from one exercise set to the next. The shorter rest time that you get in between sets is how you quickly kick your heart rate into high gear to start burning some major calories, more than you usually would.

- **Enhanced Flexibility** – Bodyweight training will force you to make use of almost every muscle in your body, sometimes pushing your body to use its full range of motion so that your joints are moving freely. This is great for loosening up all those muscles which have tightened from lack of use, and increase the mobility in your joints which then helps to improve your overall flexibility.

- **Kicks Boredom** – Repeatedly doing the same old movements and using the same equipment at the gym or at home can quickly become tedious. And boredom is the one thing you want to avoid because it can quickly become a motivation killer, which is why bodyweight training is the refreshing change in your routine that you so desperately need without even knowing it. With calisthenics exercises, there are several ways, exercises, and maneuvers that you can do which adds variety into your routine. Not only does it keep you from plateauing, but you kick boredom in the butt while pushing your fitness levels one step further each time.

- **It's Free** – Enough said. Why pay for something at the gym which you can easily do at home for free?

- **Minimal Risk of Injury** – Bodyweight training exercises are generally safe for anyone at all fitness levels because performing these exercises will force you to be aware of your body and when you're pushing too hard that you need to take it down a notch. By being more mindful and aware of your body, it minimizes your chances and risk of injury as opposed to going through the motions without thoroughly thinking and concentrating on it, which is likely to happen when relying on machines and equipment.

- **It Increases Your Strength Levels** – Being fit and physically strong is not just about how much dumbbell weight you can lift, it is also about how strong your muscles, tendons, and joints are. Bodyweight training exercises are the perfect solution to working and training your joints the way that your body is supposed to be working. Calisthenics, for example, is a great way to help develop your strength, and because bodyweight training teaches your whole body to learn to work together as a whole, it makes you stronger from within.

Chapter 2: Upper Body Workouts

Bodyweight exercises are designed to increase strength and flexibility while helping you build muscle and improve your overall fitness levels. The best part about these exercises? You can easily do them at home, or anywhere that you have space and privacy to do it!

Upper Bodyweight Workout 1 – Mountain Climbers

This move is a total body exercise which works your shoulders, upper arms, shoulders, and triceps while increasing strength and flexibility.

Step 1: Get down on the floor, supporting yourself on your arms and legs. Your legs should be stretched out behind you, toes planted firmly on the ground.

Step 2: Begin by bending your knee to bringing your right foot directly underneath your chest, keeping your other leg extended. You can start with your left foot if you prefer, either is fine.

Step 3: With your hands planted firmly on the ground (directly under your shoulders), hold your core in tight and switch legs.

Step 4: Speed this up and move your legs as fast as you can, adding a hop in between the switches.

Repeat this movement 16 times (2 sets of 8 reps). As you get stronger, increase the number of reps and your speed. For variation, instead of bending the knee directly underneath you, bringing it across your body almost as if you were trying to drive that knee into the elbow of the opposite arm. This burns the oblique muscles.

Upper Bodyweight Workout 2 – The Plyo Push-Up

Kick your regular push-up up a notch by turning up the intensity (note that you should already be able to perform a regular push-up on your hands and toes to be able to complete this move).

Step 1: Use an exercise mat for this move and position yourself in a plank position. Your arms should be straight with your palms pressed into the mat, directly underneath your shoulders as you support your upper body. Your legs are stretched out behind you, balancing on your toes.

Step 2: Bring your body down towards a push-up, elbows bent, chest lowered as far to the ground as you can go without losing form in the rest of your body.

Step 3: Now, instead of merely pushing yourself back up into the start of the push-up position, make it explosive and push up hard enough so that you're able to raise both palms slightly off the ground before landing again.

Step 4: Speed this up and get stronger into the move.

Repeat this movement 16 (2 sets of 8 reps). As you get stronger, increase the number of reps and your speed. Aim to push up higher with each explosive move too. This move is intense, so be sure to have mastered the basic push-up before attempting this variation.

Upper Bodyweight Workout 3 – Burpees

You'll be feeling the burn in your arms, chest, glutes, hamstrings and abs, even your chest with this move.

Step 1: Begin in a low-squat position, placing your palms in front of you, pressed into the floor or the mat. You should be squatting with your knees close to your hand, on either side of your palms.

Step 2: Bring your feet back one at a time into a push-up position.

Step 3: Jump back into the position that you were in Step 1, stand up tall, raising your arms above your head.

Step 4: Repeat Step 2 except this time, jump both feet back together in a seamless leap.

Repeat this movement 16 times (2 sets of 8 reps). As you get stronger, increase the number of reps and your speed. Add intensity into the workout by adding a jump instead of standing up tall.

Upper Bodyweight Workout 4– The Superman

Step 1: Begin by lying face down on a mat and your stomach. Your face should be looking down at your exercise mat during this move. Ensure that your neck remains in a neutral position throughout the move.

Step 2: Next, extend your arms up overhead, so both your arms should be right by your ears and above your head. Your legs should remain extended behind you, and your neck continues to remain in a neutral position.

Step 3: Don't lock out your legs and arms, keep them neutral along with your neck. Now, while keeping your torso still (don't move it at all), simultaneously lift both your arms and legs in an upward motion like you're trying to bend your body almost into the shape of the letter U. Your back will arch as you attempt to lift your arms and legs several inches off the floor.

Step 4: Hold this position for 5 seconds before lowering slowly back down to the ground.

Repeat this movement 24 times (3 sets of 8 reps). When lifting your arms and legs, inhale deeply and then exhale when you lower them back down to the ground.

Upper Bodyweight Workout 5– The Shoulder Tap and Plank

The move takes the regular plank bodyweight workout up a notch and targets your shoulders, arms, wrists, and core muscles at the same time.

Step 1: Begin in a full plank position, palms pressed into the ground and on your toes. Keep your belly button pulled in tight, but don't arch your back, just draw your core in tightly towards you, so it isn't drooping towards the ground.

Step 2: With your core firmly pulled in and balancing on your toes, bring your right hand up and touch your left shoulder lightly with your fingertips (in a quick tap motion) before bringing it back into the original start position. The rest of your body should remain steady during this move, keeping your legs wider apart if you need to maintain balance.

Step 3: Repeat this motion with the left hand. Alternate between both arms throughout the movement, keeping your balance steady so you're not swaying from side to side as you tap your shoulders.

Repeat this movement 24 times (3 sets of 8 reps). As you get stronger into the move, bring your feet closer and closer together until eventually, you are able to complete this move with both feet next to each other. The closer your feet are the harder it will be to maintain balance.

Upper Bodyweight Workout 6- Plank and Jacks

This move is a twist which combines planks and good old fashion jumping jacks.

Step 1: Use an exercise mat for this one to help you gauge just how far and wide you should be jumping with your feet. Get starting by lowering into a plank position. Your shoulders should be directly over your wrists for this move.

Step 2: Your body should now be in a straight line, with your feet side by side, toes pressed into the mat. Now, just like how you would do in a standing jumping jack, jump both feet out wide to the side, and then jump back in bringing both feet close together once more.

Repeat this movement 30 times (3 sets of 10 reps). As you get stronger into the move, increase the number of reps and sets you perform. For added intensity and to give your obliques a workout, jump both feet (keep them together) to the left side of your body, jump back to the start position, and then jump both feet to the right side of the body. Your feet should remain together throughout the move.

Upper Bodyweight Workout 7- Side Planks

Planks have been known to be one of those awesome moves that simultaneously work two parts of the body, your core, and your upper body strength because of how heavily you're going to rely on it to keep you balanced throughout this move.

Step 1: Start this move by lying on your side on the mat. Your right elbow should be positioned directly underneath your right shoulder. Keep your left arm raised above you, fingertips pointing towards the ceiling for this move.

Step 2: Engage your core by pulling it in tight as you then raise your body off the mat by pressing your right elbow into the floor. You are not balancing on your elbow and the sides of your feet. Keep one foot in front of the other if you need help balancing.

Step 3: Hold the plank position for 30 seconds, or 60 seconds if you can, before lowering back down and repeating the move.

Step 4: To kick it up a notch, once you are in a plank position and balancing on your elbows and sides of your feet, dip your pelvis slowly towards the floor until you're almost touching the mat before raising it back up to the start position.

Repeat this movement 12 times on each side (2 sets of 6 reps per side). As you get stronger into the move, increase the number of reps and sets you perform. For added intensity and to give your obliques a workout, jump both feet (keep them together) to the left side of your body, jump back to the start position, and then jump both feet to the right side of the body. Your feet should remain together throughout the move.

Upper Bodyweight Workout 8– Arm Circles

Arm circles are a wonderfully dynamic move that will increase mobility in those shoulder joints, the back of the arms, biceps, and triceps.

Step 1: Stand up tall, feet no wider than hip-width apart, shoulders back.

Step 2: Extend your arms out, keeping them shoulder height and parallel to the floor as you begin to make 20 small arm circles in a forward motion, both arms moving simultaneously.

Step 3: Once you've completed the movement forwards, now circle your arms in a backward motion.

If you are finding it difficult to move both arms together, alternate them one at a time, so it looks like your arms a doing the windmill. You will still be getting the full range of motion, and as you get stronger and your mobility improves, try completing wider and faster circles.

Upper Bodyweight Workout 9– Tricep Dips

Effectively work the tricep muscles, which run along the back of your upper arm from your elbow to the shoulder in one swift and efficient move known as the Tricep Dip.

Step 1: Position yourself on the floor or the mat, with your hands by your sides. Your elbows should be close in by your sides, bent at a 90-degree angle, your feet pressed firmly on the ground.

Step 2: Next, raise your body off the floor by extending your arms to propel yourself upward, raising your body into a tabletop position. Imagine that if someone were to walk in and try to balance a cup on your torso, they could before you're holding steady.

Step 3: Bend your arms again as your return to your 90-degree start position, lowering your booty until it is almost touching the matt and then left up once more.

Repeat this move 24 times (3 sets of 8 reps). As you begin to get stronger, increase the number of repetitions. For added intensity, lift one left off the floor and kick it out in front of you as you raise your body off the floor, keep it off the floor even when you lower back down and push up again. Switch legs to work both sides equally.

Upper Bodyweight Workout 10– Push-Up with Twist Rotations

As you begin to feel your body get stronger with every bodyweight movement you do, challenge your upper body even more by making your arms worker harder than ever when you add a slight variation to your regular push-up move: *a twist at the top*

Step 1: Begin in a plank position for this move. Place your feet in line with your hips, and your arms directly underneath your shoulders. Widen your arms to the sides to where you are able to complete a full-body push-up without sacrificing form.

Step 2: Lower your body towards the floor, complete the push-up and return to the start position at the top.

Step 3: When you are at the top, twist your upper body to the right, raising your right up above you with your fingertips pointing towards the ceiling. Look up at your fingertips as you do. Your pelvis and hips should hold steady, don't let it rise or fall during the twist.

Step 4: Return to plank position, complete another push-up and rotate to the left this time when you come up top.

Repeat this move 16 times (2 sets of 8 reps). As you begin to get stronger, increase the number of repetitions and your speed at which you complete the push-up and twist.

Chapter 3: Lower Body Workouts

Lower Bodyweight Workout 1 – Squats

An oldie but a goodie. Squats work multiple muscle groups at the same time, which is why they continue to remain a favorite of many fitness trainers.

Step 1: Begin by standing with your feet shoulder-width apart, knees slightly bent and make sure that your knees are not pointed over your toes.

Step 2: Place both your hands lightly behind your head on either side (right hand should be behind your right ear, left hand behind your left ear), with your fingertips lightly touching the back of your head.

Step 3: Imagine you have a chair directly behind you. Begin bending your hips and knees almost as if you were going to sit back into that chair. Make sure your knees don't extend past your toes as you attempt to sit back, that's how you know you've got the right posture for the movement. All your weight should be transferred into your heels, that is where the focus is.

Step 4: Keep your chest and shoulders upright during the sitting back movement, make sure you are not hunching forward. If it helps, try to focus on a spot or an object that is directly in front of you to keep your chest and shoulders upright. Keep your head and eyes looking straight ahead, don't stiffen your back.

Step 5: Hold the squat for 2 seconds, and the return to your standing position, using the weight in your heels to help drive your body back up.

Do this 16 times (2 sets of 8 reps). As you get stronger, increase the number of repetitions.

Lower Bodyweight Workout 2 – Jump Squats

Jump squats are a plyometric move which will cause your heart rate to spike and burn more calories as you do.

Step 1: Stand with your feet shoulder-width apart, with your hands placed firmly on either side of your hips or clasped together firmly in front of you (just like you would in a squat).

Step 2: Just as how you would sit back in a squat, repeat the same motion except this time, add an explosive jump after your squat before returning to the upright position.

Step 3: When you jump, land softly with both feet and don't lock your knees, keep them nice and relaxed, so there is no added pressure on your joint.

Beginners should aim to do this 16 times (2 sets of 8 reps). As you get stronger, increase the number of repetitions, and try to jump higher each time. Once you get stronger in the movement, you can begin doing this quicker too.

Lower Bodyweight Workout 3 – Wall Sit

Wall sits will help you strengthen your quads, hamstrings, calves, and improve your balance.

Step 1: Begin by standing with your back against the wall. Stand up tall with your shoulders back. You should not be standing too close to the wall that you find it difficult to bend your knees.

Step 2: Once you have positioned yourself comfortably, begin by raising your arms in front of you, stretched out at shoulder level. If you have better balance, you can position them on your hips.

Step 3: Slide down into a sitting position, using the wall for support, until both your knees and your hips are bent at a 90-degree angle. Continue to keep your upper back and shoulders upright (using the wall for support). Both feet should be firmly flat on the ground, and your body weight evenly distributed between both feet.

Step 4: Hold this position for 30-seconds if you are beginner before returning to an upright position. If you're more advanced, you can try holding the position for 60-seconds.

Repeat this movement 12 times (2 sets of 6 reps each). As you get stronger, increase the time intervals by 30-seconds each time.

Lower Bodyweight Workout 4 – Front Lunges

Lunges target your quads, hamstring, calves and core muscles, and they are among the most effective bodyweight exercises for toning and building muscle.

Step 1: Stand with your feet shoulder-width apart, with your hands placed firmly on either side of your hips.

Step 2: Step one foot forward (you can begin with either your right or your left). Keep your shoulders back, back tall and gaze directly in front of you to maintain your posture.

Step 3: If you step forward with your right foot first, your weight should be on the ball of your left foot. When you're ready, begin bending both knees until you have achieved a 90-degree angle.

Step 4: If you step forward with your right foot first, your knees should not extend too far past your toes when you bend at a 90-degree angle. Your upper body and gaze should remain forward, focusing on the same spot or object in front of you. This will help you maintain your balance.

Step 5: Return to standing position. You can either resume the movement with the same leg or switch legs.

Repeat this movement 32 times (16 lunges per leg). As you get stronger, increase the number of reps per leg that you do.

Lower Bodyweight Workout 5 – Jump Lunges

Just like jump squats, these jump lunges are a plyometric move which will cause your heart rate to spike and burn more calories as you do. Because this is considered a more advanced exercise, only move onto this bodyweight movement when you have mastered the basic lunge movement.

Step 1: Stand with your feet shoulder-width apart, with your hands placed firmly on either side of your hips (just like you would in a lunge).

Step 2: Step one foot forward (you can begin with either your right or your left). Keep your shoulders back, back tall and gaze directly in front of you to maintain your posture.

Step 3: If you step forward with your right foot first, your weight should be on the ball of your left foot. When you're ready, begin bending both knees until you have achieved a 90-degree angle.

Step 4: When you're in a lunge position, jump and simultaneously switch legs, landing in a jump again except this time with your opposite leg in the bent forward 90-degree position. If you started with your lunge on the right foot, when you jump and switch in the air you should now land on your left foot. Always ensure your landing is nice and quiet, with your knees soft.

Beginners should aim to do this 16 times (2 sets of 8 reps). As you get stronger, increase the number of repetitions.

Lower Bodyweight Workout 6 – Reverse Lunges

This move works your quads too, specifically the muscles in the front upper part of your legs, glutes and the adductor muscles in your inner thighs and calves.

Step 1: Stand with your feet shoulder-width apart, with your hands placed firmly on either side of your hips.

Step 2: Step one foot back (you can begin with either your right or your left). Keep your shoulders back, back tall and gaze directly in front of you to maintain your posture.

Step 3: If you step back with your right foot first, your weight should be on the ball of your left foot. When you're ready, begin bending both knees until you have achieved a 90-degree angle. Lower your back bent knee as far to the ground as you can.

Step 4: If you step back with your right foot first, you left knee should not extend too far past your toes when you bend at a 90-degree angle. Your upper body and gaze should remain forward, focusing on the same spot or object in front of you. This will help you maintain your balance.

Step 5: Return to standing position. You can either resume the movement with the same leg or switch legs.

Repeat this movement 32 times (16 lunges per leg). As you get stronger, increase the number of reps per leg that you do.

Lower Bodyweight Workout 7 – Glute Bridges

If you're having trouble squatting or lunging due to a prior injury, this workout is the next best thing you can do to still tone and strengthen your glutes, your hamstrings and your lower back at the same time.

Step 1: Lie down on your exercise mat, flat on your back. Make sure your back is not arched during this position.

Step 2: Bend your knees upright, keeping your feet firmly on the ground. Your arms should be by your sides, palms faced down, pressed into the mat for added support.

Step 3: Shift your weight to your heels while you're lying down in this position. When you're ready, raise your hips, raising the lower half of your body off the mat without arching too much.

Step 4: When you have raised your hips as high as you can go, squeeze your glute muscles at the top of the movement. Imagine you have a pencil between your glutes and you're trying to squeeze them together to keep the pencil from falling. Keep your abs tight during this movement to prevent your lower back from arching.

Step 5: Hold the position for a second or two and then return to your start position.

Repeat this movement 16 times (2 sets of 8 reps). As you get stronger, increase the number of reps and the length of your hold position at the top.

Lower Bodyweight Workout 8 – Fire Hydrant Series

This move is excellent for improving mobility, which will help you perform the other lower body exercises more effectively.

Step 1: Position yourself on your mat in a table-top position. Your palms and knees should be pressed down into the mat, your abs drawn in tight so that your back is not arched or dipping.

Step 2: When you're ready, begin by raising one leg to the side, keeping it at a 90-degree position as you do.

Step 3: Raise your bent knee to hip level by your side, hold for a second and then go back to your original start position.

Step 4: Do a couple of reps on one leg before switching legs.

Repeat this movement 32 times (2 sets of 8 reps per leg). As you get stronger, increase the number of reps.

Chapter 4: Core Training

Core Workout 1 – The Russian Twist

This sounds like a dance move, but this maneuver is going to burn your entire core section and obliques.

Step 1: Sit comfortably on the mat and bend your knees. Your heels should be about an inch away from your bottom.

Step 2: Recline back while keeping your core tight to engage your abdominal muscles. Keep your back as straight as possible and do not curve into the move. Lean as far back as you can go without compromising your form.

Step 3: Pull your hands up in front of you and clasp them together. Begin rotating and twisting from left to right and back again, keeping your core engaged the entire time.

Repeat this movement 16 times (2 sets of 8 reps). As you get stronger, lean back further into the move to engage your core even more without compromising form. For added intensity, lift one or both feet off the floor as your twist.

Core Workout 2 – The Bicycles

Do this bodyweight move known as The Bicycles to target your obliques and the rectus abdominus simultaneously.

Step 1: Lie down on the mat, pressing your lower back against the floor. Don't arch the small of your back.

Step 2: Next, place your hands behind your head, fingertips lightly touching your head. Bring your knees bent at 90-degree angles.

Step 3: Lift your upper body until you feel your shoulder blades rising off the floor. Do not pull or strain your neck during this move. As you rise, twist your upper body bringing your right elbow towards the left knee as you bend the knee in. The right leg extends out at a 45-degree angle as you do so.

Step 4: Switch sides and do the same thing on the other side.

Repeat this movement 20 times (2 sets of 10 reps). As you get stronger, increase the number of reps. For this move, it is not about how fast you can go, but about how well you can maintain your form throughout the move, so it is okay to go slow and steady as long as you're getting it right.

Upper Bodyweight Workout 3 – The Scissor Kick

Step 1: Begin by lying on your back, planning your hands on the floor either by your side or underneath your lower back if you need the extra support.

Step 2: Lift your leg a couple of inches off the ground. Lift your shoulder blades off the mat, but do now strain or pull on your neck.

Step 3: Cross your left ankle over your right, then switch and repeat.

Repeat this movement 16 times (2 sets of 8 reps). As you get stronger, increase the number of reps.

Upper Bodyweight Workout 4– The Two-Point Plank Move

This move can be tough to do if you haven't mastered the basic plank yet, because it is going to work your core muscles hard while working on your stability at the same time.

Step 1: Begin in a plank position. Hands should be directly underneath the shoulders, legs stretched out behind you as you balance on your toes.

Step 2: Once you're balanced and your torso is nice and firm, lift your left leg off the floor while simultaneously stretching out the *opposite* arm (meaning your right arm) in front of you. Hold for 5 to 10-seconds.

Step 3: Next, bring the left knee and right arm in at the same time, crossing your body as your knee and elbow meet in the middle. Release back into your start position and repeat this move on the other side.

Repeat this movement 16 times (2 sets of 8 reps each side). Increase your reps the stronger you get.

Upper Bodyweight Workout 5– The Hollow Hold

A move that looks deceptively simple, but it isn't. Because creating a strong and stable core takes hard work.

Step 1: Begin by lying on your back, with your legs stretched out in front of you. Extend your arms overhead and tighten your core.

Step 2: Focus on pressing your lower back into the mat. Now, pull your belly button in, tightening your core.

Step 3: With each inhale that you take, lift your legs, shoulders, and arms off the floor slightly. Keep your abs tight. Hold the move for 30-seconds before lowering back down.

Repeat this movement 8 times to start. As you get stronger into the move, increase the number of reps you can complete, aiming to go higher each time.

Upper Bodyweight Workout 6– The Frog Crunch

Kick your regular crunches up a notch with this intense move.

Step 1: Begin by sitting on the mat, balancing on your sit bones. You should be able to comfortably lift your feet slightly off the floor. Arms should be stretched out to the side of your body.

Step 2: As you inhale, pull your in towards your chest in the crunch motion while simultaneously bringing your arms in to hug yourself around the knees. Exhale and release back into your start position.

Repeat this movement 20 times (2 sets of 10 reps). As you get stronger into the move, increase the number of reps and sets you perform.

Upper Bodyweight Workout 7– The Roll-Down Pilates

Step 1: Sit on your mat with your arms raised above your head, knees bent, and feet pressed firmly on the grown. As you reach your arms overhead towards the ceiling, imagine like you are pulling and lengthening your spine.

Step 2: Exhale your breath and simultaneously roll down to the floor in a smooth and controlled motion. Keep your arms close by your head so that when you are on the floor, they should be directly parallel to the floor.

Step 3: Peel yourself slowly off the mat as your exhale, in a slow and controlled movement and return to your original start position.

Repeat this movement 12 times on each side (2 sets of 6 reps). As you get stronger into the move, increase the number of reps and sets you perform.

Core Workout 8– Standing Kick Crunches

Step 1: Stand up tall with your feet hip-width apart. Inhale and exhale a few times as you begin to engage your abs.

Step 2: As you inhale, lift your right leg off the floor, extending it into a kick in front of you while simultaneously bringing your left hand forward almost like you were going to touch the toes of your right leg.

Step 3: Keep your abs engaged throughout the movement, so it feels like you are crunching while you stand. Return to start position and switch legs, repeating this move on the other side.

Do this 20 times (2 sets of 10 reps each). Increase the number of reps as you get stronger.

Core Workout 9– Butterfly Crunches

Step 1: Position yourself on the mat. Bend and fold your knees out, placing the souls of your feet together. Your arms should be raised above your head, palms pressed together.

Step 2: Exhale while simultaneously bringing your hands and knees towards each other, lifting your shoulder blades and your feet off the floor. Your hands should meet your toes.

Step 3: Hold this position for 5 seconds, squeezing your abs tightly before releasing and returning to start.

Repeat this move 12 times (2 sets of 6 reps). As you begin to get stronger, increase the number of repetitions.

Core Workout 10– The Runner Crunch

Imagine you are running, except this time on the mat.

Step 1: Begin on your back. Bend your elbows at a 90-degree angle by the side of your body. Engage your core before beginning this move.

Step 2: Roll-up into a sitting position, bringing your left elbow in and twisting it towards your right knee, which you are going to raise and bend at the same time. It should look like it would if you were running.

Step 3: Lower and return to start position and repeat this move on the left side.

Repeat this move 16 times (2 sets of 8 reps). As you begin to get stronger, increase the number of repetitions and your speed.

Conclusion

Congratulations! And thank for making it through to the end of this book, let's hope it was informative and able to provide you with all of the tools you need to achieve your goals whatever they may be.

Do you see how easy it is to get a complete strength training workout for your body without the need for equipment? Calisthenics training is one of the best workouts you can do because of how easy it is to follow, and you can do it anywhere you are!

Do these strength training moves one at a time on the areas you need to work, or combine several moves for an intense strength training session and start seeing a real difference to your physique and fitness before you know it.

** Remember to use your link to claim your 3 FREE Cookbooks on Health, Fitness & Dieting Instantly

https://bit.ly/2MkqTit

CPSIA information can be obtained
at www.ICGtesting.com
Printed in the USA
LVHW082347170120
644096LV00012B/298